# Acquired Communication Impairments

EDITED BY

## Shelagh Brumfitt PhD

Professor of Speech and Language Therapy Education
Senate Award Fellow
Department of Human Communication Sciences
University of Sheffield
South Yorkshire
UK

# WILEY-BLACKWELL

A John Wiley & Sons, Ltd., Publication

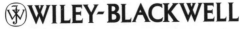

This edition first published 2010
© 2010 John Wiley & Sons Ltd

Wiley-Blackwell is an imprint of John Wiley & Sons, formed by the merger of Wiley's global Scientific, Technical and Medical business with Blackwell Publishing.

*Registered office*
John Wiley & Sons Ltd, The Atrium, Southern Gate, Chichester, West Sussex, PO19 8SQ, United Kingdom

*Editorial office*
John Wiley & Sons Ltd, The Atrium, Southern Gate, Chichester, West Sussex, PO19 8SQ, United Kingdom

For details of our global editorial offices, for customer services and for information about how to apply for permission to reuse the copyright material in this book please see our website at www.wiley.com/wiley-blackwell.

The right of the author to be identified as the author of this work has been asserted in accordance with the Copyright, Designs and Patents Act 1988.

Wiley also publishes its books in a variety of electronic formats. Some content that appears in print may not be available in electronic books.

Designations used by companies to distinguish their products are often claimed as trademarks. All brand names and product names used in this book are trade names, service marks, trademarks or registered trademarks of their respective owners. The publisher is not associated with any product or vendor mentioned in this book. This publication is designed to provide accurate and authoritative information in regard to the subject matter covered. It is sold on the understanding that the publisher is not engaged in rendering professional services. If professional advice or other expert assistance is required, the services of a competent professional should be sought.

*Library of Congress Cataloging-in-Publication Data*

Psychological well being and acquired communication impairments/[edited by] Shelagh Brumfitt.
        p.; cm.
    Includes bibliographical references and index.
    ISBN 978-0-470-06543-3
    1. Communicative disorders—Psychological aspects.  I. Brumfitt, Shelagh.
    [DNLM: 1.  Speech Disorders—psychology.  2.  Mental Health.  3.  Speech Disorders—therapy.
    4.  Speech Therapy—methods.  5.  Speech Therapy—psychology. WL 340.2 P974 2010]
    RC428.8.P79 2010
    616.85'506—dc22

                                                                2009006809


A catalogue record for this book is available from the British Library.
Set in 10/12 pt Palatino by Laserwords Pvt Ltd, Chennai, India
Printed and bound in Singapore by Fabulous Printers Pte Ltd
1    2010

# Contents

# Contributors

**Dr Jane Barton** is a consultant clinical psychologist with a special interest in psychological aspects of stroke rehabilitation. She studied at the University of Sheffield, trained in clinical psychology at the University of Leeds, and previously worked for the Medical Research Council as an occupational psychologist before commencing work in the NHS. Her main research interests currently include the process of emotional adjustment following stroke, the experience of post-traumatic stress following stroke, and driving after stroke.

**Diane Brown** qualified as a speech and language therapist in 1997 from Sheffield University. Since then she has worked as a speech and language therapist with adults in hospitals and the community, within both acute and rehabilitation settings. For the past 6 years she has worked specifically in the field of communication impairment following stroke in the Barnsley Primary Care Trust. She works as part of a multidisciplinary team on a stroke rehabilitation unit, which has allowed her to support holistically the communication needs of patients during their stay on the unit.

**Kidge Burns** first received training in solution focused brief therapy (SFBT) in 1998 and was awarded a Diploma in Solution Focused Practice in 2006. She has been at the Chelsea and Westminster Hospital as a speech and language therapist since 1998 and is the author of *Focus on Solutions; A Health Professional's Guide* (Whurr, 2005). Kidge also works as a solution focused brief therapist at a private GP clinic and is a member of the United Kingdom Association for Solution Focused Practice.

**Dr Madeline Cruice** is a Senior Lecturer and Clinical Educator at the Department of Language and Communication Science, City University London. She has taught on the undergraduate, postgraduate and master's speech and language therapy programmes on aphasia, professional studies, and issues relating to inclusion and living with disability. She has also supervised research students in the areas of quality of life, goal setting, inpatient communication and communication access. Her doctoral research investigated the relationship between communication and quality of life in older people (with/without a communication disability), and her ongoing research interests address conceptual and measurement issues in health-related quality of life and well-being. Madeline is currently leading a two year project in speech and language therapy students' clinical education experiences.

**Daniel Daneshvar** is a graduate of the Massachusetts Institute of Technology (MIT) in Cambridge, Massachusetts (USA). He received a Master's degree in medical sciences from Boston University School of Medicine, where he is currently an MD/PhD student.

**Dr Camilla Herbert** has worked in post-acute and community brain injury rehabilitation settings since qualifying as a clinical psychologist in 1988. She has worked in various locations across the UK including London, Sheffield and Leeds, and is now based in West Sussex. She continues to work within the National Health Service at the Regional Neurosciences Centre, Hurstwood Park in West Sussex, and also for the Brain Injury Rehabilitation Trust, where she is the Lead Clinician for the specialist rehabilitation centre, Kerwin Court, near Horsham.

**Mairi Knox** qualified as an occupational therapist in 1999 from the College of Ripon and York St Johns, obtaining a BSc (Hons). Since then she has worked within adult neurology services in various settings. She worked on the stroke rehabilitation unit in Barnsley for 3 years, during which time she developed an interest in enhancing the service provision for patients who experienced cognitive difficulties. Her interest in supporting patients' well-being and maintaining independence has inspired her to move into the field of vocational rehabilitation. She now works full time as a practitioner for the Condition Management Programme.

**Sabrina Poon** is a graduate of Yale University in New Haven, Connecticut. Following her undergraduate degree she worked as a research assistant at the Boston University School of Medicine's Alzheimer's Disease Clinical and Research Program. She is currently a medical student at Vanderbilt School of Medicine in Nashville, Tennessee (USA).

**Dr Shonagh Scott** is a principal clinical psychologist with a special interest in psychological aspects of stroke and in the mental health of older people. She studied at Edinburgh University and completed her clinical training at Sheffield University before joining the NHS. Her clinical and research interests include: psychological adjustment to stroke, psychotherapeutic groups for people with dementia, staff training and supervision.

**Dr Robert A. Stern** is Associate Professor of Neurology at Boston University School of Medicine, where he is also Co-Director of the Alzheimer's Disease Clinical and Research Program, and Co-Director of the Center of the Study of Traumatic Encephalopathy. Dr Stern has published on various aspects of assessment and is the senior author of several neuropsychological and neuropsychiatric tests and instruments. His primary areas of funded research include Alzheimer's disease, driving and dementia, thyroid–brain relationships, and the long-term effects of repetitive concussion in athletes. Dr Stern has received several National Institutes of Health and other local grants, has published over 200 journal articles, chapters and abstracts, and is a Fellow of both the American Neuropsychiatric Association and the National Academy of Neuropsychology. He is an Associate Editor of the *Journal of Neuropsychiatry and Clinical Neurosciences* and is on the Editorial Board of *Archives of Clinical Neuropsychology*.

**Dr Shirley A. Thomas** is a Lecturer in Rehabilitation Psychology at the University of Nottingham. She completed a PhD in psychology and the topic of her doctoral thesis was identifying factors relating to emotional distress after stroke. Her current research interest includes the assessment and management of mood problems in people with communication problems.

## About the editor

**Shelagh Brumfitt** is a professor of Speech and Language Therapy Education and has a long-standing interest in approaches to psychosocial aspects of aphasia and other communication impairments. With co-author (Professor Paschal Sheeran, University of Sheffield) she developed the VASES, one of the first measures of self-esteem using picture material as an aid to comprehension in a self-esteem scale. From 1997 to 1999 she was Chair of the Academic Board of the Royal College of Speech and Language Therapists and was awarded the Honours of the Royal College of Speech and Language Therapists in 2006. In 2007 she was awarded a University of Sheffield Award for Sustained Excellence in Teaching and Learning.

# Foreword

There is a growing interest among health professionals throughout the developed world in the emotional and affective problems faced by people with neurogenic communication problems and their relatives, and this interest is likely to increase. Speech and language therapists and pathologists working with people with neurogenically caused communication problems have a particular concern, because as a group they probably spend more time with this population than do other health professionals. The concern has significantly increased in recent years reflecting the increased appreciation that the emotional impact of brain damage and communication impairment can have a devastating effect on the individual and their relatives and friends.

However, it is a mistake to think that we have only recently become aware of emotional consequences of brain damage. As early as 1904 Meyer recognised that brain-damaged individuals experienced particular emotional reactions. Babinski in 1922 originally described the *indifference reaction* he associated with right hemisphere damage, and in 1939 Kurt Goldstein, a pioneer in many aspects of aphasia, described the *catastrophic reactions* often experienced by those with left hemisphere damage. Guido Gainotti went on to examine such left–right differences more systematically, in his seminal study of 1972. Such work emphasises that the emotions we feel are embedded in the workings of our brains and nervous systems.

More recent work has shown that the emotional impact of brain damage can be either a direct result of damage to the electrochemical underpinnings of emotions in the brain or a more indirect, reactive response to devastating life events, like a stroke, head injury and other neurological disease processes: these separate causes are sometimes called *primary* and *secondary* reactions. While it is often difficult to determine in clinical practice whether an observed emotional response is direct or indirect, or both, in the senses described above, there are indications emerging that the different causes may respond better to different management approaches. So it would be a mistake to dismiss this division as merely of theoretical relevance.

However, the increasingly recognised emotional impact of communication impairments following brain damage, and their negative effects on response to rehabilitation effort, do not appear to have resulted in sufficiently increased or enhanced services aimed at their management. There are many in the community experiencing such emotional reactions who have 'slipped through the net', such that there was a 'net' to catch them in the first place. It is still the case that there is little psychological help and support or counselling available for those affected, and almost none for the relatives who are known to bear so much of the burden for the years following an initial neurological incident.

This volume, devoted to the psychological well-being of people with acquired communication problems, is therefore particularly welcome. Professor Shelagh Brumfitt is very well known and well respected for her pioneering work in this area and has extensive experience in the topic. A particularly welcome feature of this book is the mixture of professional perspectives that she has brought to the topic of psychological well-being in people with communication problems. She has herself been a pioneer of interdisciplinary work between speech and language therapists and clinical psychologists, and this is a particularly welcome and unique feature of the collection of practically useful chapters. The perspectives and expertise of speech and language therapists, occupational therapists and clinical psychologists are represented within the chapters of the book. Topics range across the main issues for the field: how do we validly and reliably recognise and assess emotions in people who have communication difficulties and what approaches can we use to manage these devastating conditions? The answers are by no means all in. Problems remain for assessment and for management. It is often said that the best way to find out how someone is feeling is to ask them, and, by necessity, so much of the basic research that has been done with aphasic participants has been with those whose aphasia is relatively mild. However, a number of chapters explore the wide range of available approaches to assessment, several minimally dependent on verbal abilities. Similarly, for management, issues still remain concerning pharmaceutical intervention versus a more psychological one, and these different approaches are explored. A genuine interdisciplinary approach involving medical and therapeutic workers, where drug treatments are closely monitored and managed, and counselling, group therapies and other 'talking' therapies are made more widely available for patients and relatives, is a challenge for all those concerned.

Shelagh Brumfitt and her contributors deserve congratulations for their work, which I believe provides valuable and practical knowledge to help us face the challenges posed by the emotional impact of neurogenic communication problems, and much needed help and support for the psychological well-being of people with acquired communication problems and their relatives.

Chris Code
Foundation Professor of Communication Sciences and Disorders
University of Sydney
Visiting Professor at School of Psychology, University of Exeter
November 2008

# Preface

This book arose out of a long-standing interest and commitment to the emotional and psychological needs of people with acquired communication impairment. A further motivation arose from seeing the growth in the evidence base for this subject. This is an appropriate time to put together material from some of the key authors in this field.

I moved into work as a speech and language therapist with people with acquired communication impairments in 1976. My job was based around a neurosurgical unit in a large hospital in the UK, and I covered all the referrals from any ward in the hospital. The patients were people who had suffered road traffic accidents, other traumatic head injuries, stroke and neurological diseases, and anyone else who happened to come into the hospital and was found to be having difficulty with communication. At the time professionals such as speech and language therapists and clinical psychologists were rare people. The hospital had only ever had two speech and language therapists, in total. If my memory is correct, I was the third and while I was there another speech and language therapist was appointed to come in for a few days each week.

The neurosurgical unit was a significant learning experience for me. Of course, I 'knew' that people my own age could have strokes or be involved in road traffic accidents. But by being on the ward every day I was soon confronted with the extent of the impact these conditions had. There was the child who had run into the road and been hit by a car, and had severe dysarthria. A young woman, who had severe headaches and eventually gone to a doctor to find she needed emergency surgery for an aneurysm, was left with aphasia and hemiplegia at the age of 21. Then the academic who had a sudden cerebral haemorrhage which resulted in aphasia. His academic subject specialism became very difficult to communicate. To a speech and language therapist at the time, the therapeutic challenges were immense. Services were much less sophisticated than they are now and the understanding of the conditions much less advanced. It is probably impossible to communicate to new health professionals how much we were expected to think of our own solutions. Some important aspects of practice were just emerging, such as more standardised guidelines for therapy. The emergence of theoretical models, such as cognitive neuropsychology, to understand specific conditions was beginning. We had no computers.

But in many of the sorts of units just described there were good opportunities for discussions with other professionals, and clinical psychologists were often very interested in the same types of conditions. There is a natural link in that many patients experience extreme losses of their skills and feel the emotional consequences of this. However, the specific complexity in this situation is around the management and expression of emotion and the impact of limited communication. It is this challenge that has confronted both professional groups, where both needed to know how to assess these conditions and work out helpful intervention strategies.

The focus of this book is to provide a text that brings together the gathering evidence about the area of psychological well-being in people with communication impairments. It will serve as a textbook to guide students who will work as health professionals and it will serve as one of the first books to bring together a multidisciplinary approach to this critical subject. All of the authors have direct professional experience of people with acquired communication impairments and have been invited to contribute to the book because of their recognised skills in clinical management and academic inquiry.

There are two important clinical areas to examine in relation to this. Firstly, the book aims to look at approaches to assessment of the subjective experiences of a person with an acquired communication impairment; and secondly, it aims to develop an understanding of relevant intervention approaches. The book focuses on both of these aspects although it is important to stress that this material is not comprehensive. This topic is a growing international topic and research is being conducted now that will influence approaches in the future.

Many of the chapters in the book seek to address the practical application of this knowledge base and for that reason include sample case studies to highlight the discussions. The book includes chapters on approaches to assessment of anxiety and depression, the impact of brain injury and the role of quality of life issues in acquired communication impairments. There is a chapter on the role of an assessment of mood and one on the role of self-esteem. Examples of specific assessments can be found in these chapters and these are linked to case studies describing the management of sample patients. Intervention approaches at different time points in the patient journey are also presented and guidelines for use in practice are provided in these chapters.

This subject has grown substantially since my early years as a practitioner, and the experience of patients has improved considerably. There is diversity in people with acquired communication impairments and there is diversity in the professional approaches to management of their well-being. However, this book has aimed to bring together some commonalities that form a sound evidence base from which the student or health professional can develop their knowledge and skills.

Shelagh Brumfitt

# 1   Introduction

## Shelagh Brumfitt

## Why is this topic of importance?

The subjective experience of people with acquired communication impairments has been of concern to health professionals for a long time, with contributions to knowledge coming from a range of professional fields, most particularly from Speech and Language Therapy and from Clinical Psychology. This book creates the opportunity to discuss these contributions. It aims to bring together material on psychological well-being from the academic literature and to discuss how it may be applied to professional practice with people who have acquired communication impairments. It allows the perspectives of different professional groups to contribute to this area of work and creates opportunities for working across boundaries in the healthcare context.

Although it has been widely recognised in the literature that people with acquired communication impairments have intense emotions and distress about their situation, specific methods for helping have only emerged slowly. Various influencing factors have affected progress. For example, aphasic speakers may often be excluded from research into psychological well-being, if they are viewed as unable to comply with the data collection because of their linguistic difficulties. Typically, the data collection would involve a questionnaire, and the severely impaired aphasic speaker may find this too complex to respond to. This has therefore limited the research evidence. In addition, methods for analysing the psychological or emotional responses of participants with communication impairment have been unavailable until recently (Gainotti, 1997). Our understanding of emotional reactions to brain damage has had to be drawn from the non-communicatively impaired population, and this theoretical framework may not transfer well.

For people who experience a stroke, brain injury or a progressive neurological illness, the loss of communicative ability can be a shattering experience. Ordinary everyday conversations may become impossible, complex discussions are out of reach, and access to a normal social life and employment may be difficult. Although there is an abundance of material about how to describe the different types of communication impairments, the way that loss of communication relates to psychological well-being still needs to be brought into a wider academic and professional arena. As Tanner and Gerstenberger (1988) state, 'a person's psychological status cannot be separated from the neuropathology of speech and language' (p. 84).

By far the greatest amount of research has been done into aphasia and the depressive reaction (Code and Herrmann, 2003). It is not clear why this should be, other than clinicians observe depressive reactions in aphasic speakers and are motivated to seek solutions. It does not really explain why there is so little research into anxiety impairments and acquired communication impairments, or why subjective experiences of people with progressive conditions have been so under-researched in comparison. Recently De Wit *et al.* (2008) examined over 500 participants who were post-stroke and not specifically people with acquired communication impairments. In this large multicentre study the results showed that the prevalence of anxiety was 22–25% and depression 24–30% during the first 6 months post-stroke. The authors noted that anxiety was almost as common as depression. This result may provide useful guidance for understanding the prevalence in the communicatively impaired population.

The purpose of this book is not to examine the nature and description of acquired communication impairments nor is it to focus on the social model of disability and how this challenges traditional therapeutic methods. These aspects are already addressed in other formats. This book aims to look specifically at current thinking on psychological well-being and how it may be managed in these populations. Few books look at this critical field although the needs of this population are great. It is intended that the multidisciplinary format will draw from a wide variety of sources and allow the reader a greater understanding than with a uniprofessional approach.

## Types of acquired communication impairments

The main types of communication impairments that affect people with acquired aetiologies are language based or related to motor speech difficulties.

### Aphasia (often termed 'dysphasia')

One of the most common causes of aphasia is stroke, but this language impairment can be seen in brain injury and cerebral tumour (Kolb and Whishaw, 2003). Acquired disordered communication, not aphasia, can be seen in other conditions such as dementia or traumatic brain injury (Royal College of Speech and Language Therapists, 2005). Aphasia is an acquired condition and occurs because of a focal lesion to the dominant hemisphere of the brain. The key symptoms focus on the impaired ability to understand spoken or written language and the impaired ability to use spoken and written language. The symptoms will vary in degree of severity across these modalities and there may be a great amount of individual variation in how these communicative impairments present. Essentially, aphasia can show a breakdown in any of the linguistic domains: syntactic, pragmatic, morphological, lexical, semantic, phonological and orthographic. It is important to note that these domains do not function independently: associations between them can be observed in different forms and these will be individual to the patient. There may also be difficulties with non-linguistic communication, such as gesture or drawing. Diagnosis of aphasia can be complicated by the presence of other conditions that may co-occur, such as apraxia of speech (apraxia of speech occurs as a result of disturbances of motor programming of movements for speech, including selection, programming and control of movements (RCSLT, Communicating Quality, 2006).

The most important development in the understanding of aphasia has been the application of a cognitive neuropsychological framework (Shallice, 1988) for explaining language breakdown. This model permits understanding of function in cognition and language impairment. Clinically, it allows detailed assessments of language that reveal specific modules or routes between modules. This has allowed a much closer understanding of where language breaks down in the individual and therefore creates opportunities to focus on specific areas of deficit more easily. Furthermore the direction for assessment is primarily on the description of the individual profile rather than on group patterns of aphasia. This approach to understanding aphasia has been a significant direction in research, from building on original understanding (Ellis and Young, 1988) to applying the model to assessment (Kay, Coltheart and Lesser, 1992; Byng, Kay, Edmundson and Scott, 1996). Approaches to intervention have been extensively developed (Howard and Franklin, 1988; Whitworth, Webster and Howard, 2005). Using the social model of disability as a framework to understand the individual response to being an aphasic speaker has also been applied through work on the psychosocial effects (Code, 2003; Parr, 2004; van der Gaag et al., 2005). Research into the emotional consequences of aphasia has been reviewed in relation to rehabilitation (Code and Herrman, 2003).

### Acquired dysarthria

Now commonly described in the plural, acquired dysarthrias are a group of motor speech disorders that result from damage to the neurological control systems governing the movements and integration of the muscles that control speech production. The symptoms will be directly linked to where the damage has occurred in the central or peripheral nervous system, and therefore the physical components involved in respiration, voicing, articulation or prosody can be implicated. These components also have other functions, of course, so the impact may extend beyond speech and typically can include other, non-verbal, activities involving the vocal tract, such as chewing, swallowing or facial expression. The degree of functional limitation can vary widely, however, from a very mild paresis of the facial muscles, with similar relatively minor speech limitations, to severe limitations of speech, voice and swallowing. (For further information, see The Stroke Association's website: http://www.stroke.org.uk/information/all_about_stroke/rehabilitation/communication/dysarthria_and.html.)

Yorkston, Beukelman, Strand and Bell (1999) describe two main groupings of acquired dysarthria. The first group is caused by stroke or traumatic brain injury and is characterised by an acute onset, followed by a period of recovery, which will later become a stable, long-term level of functional limitation. The other group is described as 'progressive/degenerative'; this includes conditions such as Parkinsons's disease (see the Parkinson's Disease Society website: http://www.parkinsons.org.uk/default.aspx?page=7237) and motor neurone disease (see the website of the Motor Neurone Disease Association: http://www.mndassociation.org/), where the pattern of the dysarthria may follow a fairly typical pattern of gradual limitation that follows the progression of the other physical symptoms (Patten, 1996). A slightly different pattern occurs with multiple sclerosis (see the website of the Multiple Sclerosis Society: http://www.mssociety.org.uk/), which Yorkston, Beukelman, Strand and Bell (1999) identify as 'progression/remission', again following the pattern of the physical symptoms.

### Brain injury

Camilla Herbert, in Chapter 3, describes the communicative impairments that may result from brain injury. Because of the nature of brain injury, the communicative symptoms can vary greatly (see the Headway website: http://www.headway.org.uk/). Types of aphasia may occur and symptoms of dysarthria may also be present depending on the site of the lesion. Further communicative difficulties are often seen including difficulties in the pragmatic aspect of communication, such as turn taking in conversation, maintenance of a topic in conversation, interpreting subtleties (such as the use of analogies in language, differences between sarcasm and serious statement) and keeping up with other speakers when the conversation is fast paced. There may be reductions of verbal fluency, word coherence and content aspects of language such as relevance of word choice (Royal College of Speech and Language Therapists, 2005).

### Progressive forms of aphasia

Originally defined by Mesulam (2001), primary progressive aphasia (PPA) is described as gradual and progressive deterioration in various components of language function (word finding disturbances). It can proceed to impair grammatical structure and comprehension of semantics. It usually begins with mild word finding difficulties and ends in its most severe form, with little meaningful use of language. This progression is generally considered to exist within the context of preserved other abilities such as memory, visual processing and personality, so that all difficulties within the first two years are associated with the language impairment and not other factors. There is debate within the literature about the form of other types of progressive language impairments, which present as either non-fluent aphasia or semantic dementia. There is much variation in the diagnosis and management of this condition.

What is important to note about the range of communication impairments that are acquired is that their presentation will be of an individual nature. Prior to the onset of the illness the experience of the individual is of knowing only that communication is easy and straightforward. At the onset of the illness, the capacity for easy communication is lost and it is this personal struggle with the loss of a previous skill that creates the personal difficulties for the individual. Our knowledge and understanding about the range of communication impairments grows all the time, but it is the emotional consequences of the loss of communication that must be understood more fully (Royal College of Physicians, 2005; Royal College of Speech and Language Therapists, 2005). It is likely that more understanding of this will follow in the future as the assessment and diagnostic methodologies become more sophisticated and the number of health professionals with specialist skills in these conditions increases.

## Psychological well-being

Although a broad concept, the definition of psychological well-being usually includes levels of mood and mood disturbances, such as depression and anxiety. Signs and symptoms of depression include feelings of a low mood for a long period of time, feeling irritable, difficulties in concentration, tiredness, inability to derive pleasure, feeling numb, empty and hopeless, sleep disturbances, feelings of guilt and negative thoughts. Symptoms of anxiety include both psychological and physical effects. The key physical components include feelings of tightness in chest, nausea, loss of appetite, butterfly feelings in stomach, pounding heart, muscle tension and sweating. The psychological features include fearful anticipation, inability to concentrate, constant worrying, heightened alertness, sleep disturbance and a strong link with depression. Both conditions have further specific features such as bipolar depressive symptoms or severe panic disorder, but these are generally not included in relation to symptoms associated with acquired brain damage. Self-esteem or self-worth is usually considered within the broad concept of well-being, with the most important difference being that depression and anxiety have a medical diagnosis and self-esteem does not. Typically, people who are depressed will have low self-esteem, and, probably, people with high self-esteem are unlikely to be depressed (Brumfitt and Sheeran, 1999). Further discussion of these conditions will be developed in subsequent chapters.

## Factors affecting psychological well-being in the person with acquired communication impairment

In order for the authors in this book to consider the psychological effects of acquired communication impairment, it is necessary to consider contributing factors. Most authors will agree that the specific communication impairment itself will not account for the whole of the psychological impact. Other aspects will influence how the individual reacts to the loss of communication capacity. Gainotti (1997, p. 635) notes that the emotional impairments associated with becoming aphasic are complex to disentangle, and include the type of brain injury, the effects upon cognitive, communicative and motor function, the premorbid personality and behavioural factors, and the patient's own social context.

Thus, even though people with acquired communication impairments share a common diagnosis, they remain individuals who have different responses to the effects of the brain damage. In terms of psychological well-being particularly, there will be differences influenced by the context in which the individual lives. These aspects deserve some recognition now, at the start of the book, to highlight their relevance.

The complexities are represented in Figure 1.1, which shows the range of factors influencing the individual's personal experience of acquired communication impairment. Broadly, these can be subdivided into internal and external factors.

### Internal factors

These relate to the individual person and include the demographic profile as well as the nature of the physical condition. Further, the type of the communication impairment and particularly its impact upon the individual's life will be internal and unique to the person. There will also be variation in how a person feels and how well they can communicate their inner feelings. This may have a direct influence on accuracy of diagnosis and whether professionals offer psychological support, as the person who can communicate that they feel sad and distressed is more likely to gain support and help than the person who cannot make this clear. Thus, difficulties in communicating feelings may be part of the overall communication impairment profile or there may be specific challenges in talking about feelings that may influenced by family and cultural tradition. An individual may have grown up in a family where talking about feelings was seen as something weak or shameful, and therefore to express distress in a health context may not be part of the individual's typical behaviour. Past history of mood disturbances can also influence how likely an individual is to experience this as part of their condition, and

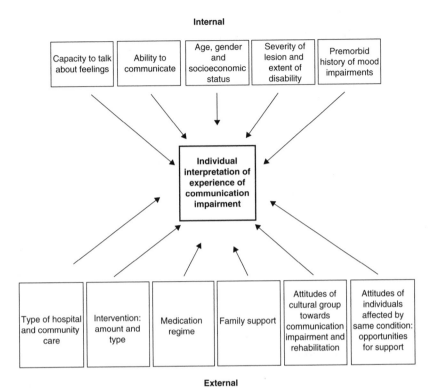

**Figure 1.1** Factors influencing the individual's personal experience of acquired communication impairment.

it may be that the individual's response to the stress of communicative loss reflects how emotional responses developed at an earlier stage in the individual's life. Clearly, a tendency to mood disorder will have implications for the coping abilities of the patient after the acute illness stage, and this is discussed by Barton in Chapter 7 on interdisciplinary approaches to managing stroke. A family history of mood disorder is also a possible marker for future difficulties for the patient.

### External factors

These include the features of the context in which the individual experiences the condition, and can include social and attitudinal aspects of other people who may be close to the individual, or broader aspects such as cultural understandings of disability. These factors will also include type and nature of healthcare and therapeutic interventions, which may vary in amount and when offered in relation to the time since onset of the condition. Interventions may or may not include direct work on psychological well-being. The medication regimes may also have an effect upon mood in a positive or negative way. Family support will also be relevant, where one individual may have longstanding support from a spouse whereas another may be isolated, living alone and unable to access services easily.

Because of the variation in how the individual interprets and copes with communication impairment, the management of the individual and the support required will have to be adapted to special needs. For some individuals the environment may be the aspect that can be changed. For other individuals, attitudes of their cultural group may have the biggest impact upon their experience of coping. Significant developments in the understanding of social influences on the person with acquired communication impairments have been made in recent years, which have changed the course of intervention approaches (see the Connect website: http://www.ukconnect.org/index.aspx; Pound *et al.*, 2000; Parr *et al.*, 1997; Duchan and Byng, 2004; Parr, Duchan and Pound, 2004). The social model has challenged current assumptions about approaches to therapy and the increased awareness about the environment, including health professionals' own attitudes to therapy. In recent years there have been huge shifts in attitudes towards enabling patients to cope positively with acquired communication impairments and not be stigmatised. Other factors may include the experience of healthcare and rehabilitation, which may not be available easily or for long enough or be sufficiently specialised. This may be an external influence over which the individual has little control. Different approaches to healthcare may mean that the individual remains isolated from other people who have similar conditions and experiences. Volunteer services may provide these opportunities, or they may be accessed through professional health settings.

## Medication

It is not the brief of this book to recommend appropriate medication for these populations, but it is worth noting current views about its use. Until recently, very little has been written about the specific use of medication in the treatment of psychological well-being in people with acquired communication impairments. The Royal College of Physicians (2005), in their published guidelines on depression following acquired brain injury, evaluate the role of antidepressants. Particular note is made of the fact that none of the existing antidepressant agents has a UK licence that specifically approves use for acquired brain injury. So that in spite of the recognition of psychological responses to acquired brain injury, very little development has taken place to enhance psychological support by medication for this group of people. Clearly, this needs to change. Apart from the obvious need to help individuals feel more psychologically stable, the potential impact upon responses to rehabilitation must not be underestimated. The individual who is depressed is potentially more likely to feel unmotivated to engage fully with rehabilitation approaches.

Direct medical advice to prescribing clinicians is, however, provided in the published report (2005), which recommends the use for depression of agents from the main classes of relevant medications. These are broadly: selective serotonin re-uptake inhibitors (SSRIs), such as fluoxetine, citalopram and escitalopram; and other antidepressant agents, which are recommended for use as 'second line' drugs when SSRIs have not been effective. These have not been fully tested in the context of acquired brain injury. Doctors are recommended to use a specific SSRI such as citalopram or sertraline as the most relevant medication. Anderson (1997) also recommends the use of SSRIs, particularly citalopram, based on a series of studies during the first year post-stroke. Anderson recommends this drug for patients with post-stroke pathological crying. The Royal College of Physicians' (RCP's) report also notes the untested use of St John's wort and its possible use with acquired brain damage. The current guidelines state that patients must be monitored throughout any medication regime for treatment of depression. One criticism of past practice included in this publication is that antidepressants have been prescribed routinely in haste and that this may not be appropriate for all.

### Consideration of further aspects

There remains some debate about whether subjective experiences of well-being are due purely to brain damage (i.e. site of lesion, severity and nature) or to secondary reactions that are emotional responses to the predicament the individual experiences. One confusing presentation in people with acute acquired communication impairments brought about by brain lesions is a set of symptoms that have been given different labels in recent times: emotional lability or post-stroke emotionalism or pathological crying (Anderson, 1997). These symptoms usually include rapid changes in mood where very strong emotions are shown such as extreme crying or laughing or even an increase in anger. The expression of these emotions may not reflect the true feelings that the individual has, but are associated instead with damage to the part of the brain that affects emotional awareness and emotional control. The presentation of the feeling is not necessarily associated with an emotionally significant thought or context. It may be the case that thoughts of close family may bring on these emotions but the behaviour may also be associated with common everyday interactions such as making arrangements about meals. Anderson (1997) reported that post-stroke pathological crying is more common than generally understood and quotes studies where 20% of patients during the first year post-stroke have shown these symptoms. In severe cases Anderson (1997) reports episodes of post-stroke pathological crying as occurring up to 100 times a day. These may be very difficult symptoms for the individual to cope with. Furthermore, potential difficulties are created for the professional in making an accurate diagnosis of true depression or pathological crying. Pathological crying or lability may be seen in other neurological conditions, such as motor neurone disease and multiple sclerosis.

## Effects of psychological well-being on communication

Although primarily this discussion is about the effect of the communication impairment on well-being, there is a small literature that describes the effects of low well-being on speech characteristics. For example, there has been some research into the effect on communicative behaviours when a person is experiencing depression. In terms of depression, communication shows a reduced speech tempo, with a listless flat manner and reduced volume, stress and rhythm. There may be increased pausing. Language is described as being limited to essential communications about everyday matters. 'Depressed or low mood restricts language and renders it colourless and limited' (France, 2001, p. 76).

Auerbach and Karow (2003) discuss issues associated with assessment of mood and affect in patients with neurological disorders. They alert the reader to the factors that may influence understanding of different conditions. For example, the neurological condition may limit how well the individual can communicate feelings, and this is potentially a risk situation if the individual is severely depressed but unable to express this. Auerbach and Karow (2003) refer to four factors that can influence this situation. Firstly, the loss of functions resulting from the brain damage will create a natural response to loss that will make the individual sad and possibly depressed. Secondly, the lesion itself can affect the individual's behaviour, as in people with Parkinson's disease where changes to movement abilities may create impairments in communicating by gesture or using facial expression. Alternatively, some neurological conditions may make the individual appear as if they are distressed, as in the case of emotional lability, when in fact they do not have a mood disorder. People with some forms of neurological disease may experience limitations of cognitive function so that normal or typical expression of emotion may emerge in a more atypical form, as in ritualistic behaviours or self-harm. Finally, the role of medication must not be overlooked in this area, because medications can affect mood and behaviour. Auerbach and Karow (2003) suggest that abilities should be evaluated in order to determine whether the individual does experience legitimate emotional disturbance. They advocate that the individual ability to recognise facial and gestural expression and speech prosody should be investigated. In terms of expressive non-verbal abilities they state that the individual's capacity to use facial expression, affective speech prosody, gesture and general motor activity needs evaluation. In relation to verbal abilities, they recommend assessment of comprehension of emotional words and humour, and for expression the use of emotional language and humour should be investigated. To some extent this framework can be applied to the context of people with communication impairments, although clearly the specific difficulties in communication would need further examination. This is elaborated further by Stern, Daneshvar and Poon in Chapter 6.

Gravell and France (1991) use the analogy of a vicious circle where poor communication leads to depression, and depression makes the individual less good at talking, which then can lead to a further reduction in mood. The individual may lose communicative abilities through acquired brain damage and may experience distress at this loss. Distress leading to depression can result in communicative changes. Thus the patient may have communicative difficulties due to aphasia and secondary communicative difficulties due to depression. This may be of importance to the practitioner in terms of differential diagnosis.

## Personal descriptions

There are many personal descriptions of acquired communication impairments in the literature (Moss, 1972; Newborn, 1997; Mackay, 2003). Individuals with acquired communication impairments are confronted by their changed communication abilities in almost every interaction they have with others. In his exploration into the social construction of aphasia, Mackay (2003, p. 825) describes the person with aphasia who 'lives surrounded by aphasia in every part of her/his life'.

Professionals involved with people with communication impairments are always concerned about how the individual responds to the changes in communication ability. What is often unclear is whether certain feelings are common to all or whether these feelings differ between individuals. Does everybody feel the same? Do feelings change over time? How do you come to understand yourself as a person with an acquired communication impairment? Personal accounts are essential to the knowledge base as it is only with the reports of subjective experience that professionals and the general public can gain a good understanding of the implications of loss of communicative abilities. There are now many personal accounts that reflect the feelings of the individual with acquired communication impairment, and the historical accounts discussed earlier highlight the variations in how people respond to this situation.

Brumfitt (1989) reports the personal experiences of a university lecturer who became aphasic, with a commentary on his struggle to adapt to his changed circumstances. The patient reported his distress on realising his academic skills were now much more limited and how this affected all aspects of his life. In a comment that revealed his inner struggle he said: 'it's so hard trying to become a person again' (Brumfitt, 1989, p. 5). One question posed by this report is about the specific effect on the identity of people with language loss compared with those who experience brain damage with no impact on language. Is the struggle to make sense of the situation more problematic with a language impairment? Intuitively it seems that this must be so. Individuals need language and potentially, inner language, to be able to make sense of their situation, and so with limited language abilities the adjustment to change is more challenging.

## Identity

The recognition of loss of identity during the recovery stages has been frequently reported in other health conditions. Bury (1991) describes the 'biographical disruption' that occurs at the onset of chronic illness where the known identity and context experienced by the individual is lost. Charmaz (1995) has focussed on the changes to identity in people with chronic illness, and described the interaction between bodily changes and identity. As individuals adapt, either to a recovery process or a set of bodily changes that are deteriorations in capacity; the sense of who they are has to move with that process. Goals and aspirations become adjusted to what is possible, but the process of being able to adapt and cope with the changed self can be very painful. There has been some debate in the academic literature on stroke, about whether the individual creates a new sense of self because of the disruption; or whether the individual views the effects of the stroke as separate to the pre- and post-stroke sense of self which, remains a coherent thread (Faircloth *et al.*, 2004). Parr *et al.* (1997) refer to this loss of identity in aphasia, where the onset of aphasia disrupts the continuous life course of the individual. Furthermore, the interaction between the experience of the communication impairment and society's reaction to it has been recognised through the work of various authors (Jordan and Kaiser, 1996).

## Personal experiences

Some examples of personal experiences are included here. They reveal the personal struggle to cope with the unexpected development of an acquired communication impairment.

### Aphasia

M qualified as a doctor in 1978, having been a successful medical student. She had a special interest in dermatology, and worked in the local hospital clinics as well as being a partner in a city centre general practice. In 1994 she was diagnosed with a space-occupying lesion (origin undetermined) and underwent neurosurgery. She was left with a degree of aphasia. In Box 1.1 she recalls her early experiences after the surgery.

### Box 1.1   M's early experiences after neurosurgery

'You didn't know whether anything was going to come out...you knew you were thinking but whether you were going to be able to express yourself...and it was case of the words were there but they didn't seem to be in any order and they didn't seem to be stored properly. It was as if somebody had gone into the library and thrown all the books in the air.'

'And the number of cups of hospital coffee I ended up with because I said yes rather than no. The number of people I confused and said good morning to; you know any greeting would have come out. Not particularly 'good morning' it could have been 'bye bye'. The words were there but I couldn't guarantee what I was getting.'

M was able to describe her experiences in relation to well-being in a vivid way. Initially the interviewer asked her about whether healthcare staff acknowledged her feelings and offered her guidance or medication.

M: 'No... I think I was seen as someone who had had a traumatic episode in my health and I ought to feel that I was lucky to be alive and to be thankful'.

Box 1.2 contains her further comments on the loss of her well-being.

### Box 1.2    Further insights from M into her loss of well-being

'Very very upset. Words had always been top priority to me... er I suppose one would say it was depression it was the big black hole you thought you were never going to get out of... I was very tired and even now if I work with words I'm much more tired than if I do physical work. And it was I suppose part of the nature of the beast... there's no point in crying because it doesn't do anything apart from give you a red nose but em there was the feeling it would have been better to just die rather than have the hassle of trying to fight back.'

'It feels it and er it's I suppose more then anything else it is the fact... I was there, I was willing, I wanted to get better, there wasn't any point at staying at the level I was at. I either had to top myself in my mindset... or I had to get better...'

'There are some times when to express your extreme despair you just want to howl you can quite see why the women keen ('to lament the dead', Irish Gaelic term, *Collins English Dictionary*) after a bereavement... there are just no words how despairing you are and I think that is the worst aspect that nobody actually acknowledges that that is where you are starting from and that's where you are going back to if things go wrong.'

'It's at times just so difficult to try and explain how demoralised you feel'.

The aphasia had a major impact on M's everyday life in relation to her career and social life. Her comments about this are in Box 1.3.

## Box 1.3 How aphasia impacted M's career and social life

'I had a bit of a paralysis but I have sorted it out over time. But I can cope. The ability to read had gone as well. There is no enjoyment in watching TV if you can't make out the nuances or anything else. And when I wanted to write a letter of thank you to the nursing staff and I wanted to spell the word 'whilst' ... I had 14 different attempts and not one of them was the right one. My mother kept them. Basically once she had shown me it ... yes it was obvious, but even now, if I try if there's something that you need to sound out phonetically ... I don't understand why. It's almost as if the connection isn't there.'

'I had to retire because basically I hadn't got the health to go back in because they needed me back in two years and it was a city centre practice ... a lot of hands on and so I was retired.'

'Sometimes I've paid to go to the theatre and I can't make out what's going on the stage and you're hesitant to say anything as to whether they're not being very clear with the diction or whether it's your filters which have gone and so you find yourself very diffident about criticising anything which might be bad in case it's your competence ... enjoy it or understand it. I used to have a couple of foreign languages but they've gone completely.'

'Also if there is a lot of outside noise and even on a good day if I was trying to have this conversation with you and there was someone with a loud voice here then there's no way I can hear myself think. So that is major problem now ... if there are other noises then the concentration isn't good enough to shut them out'.

M was asked to describe other people's attitudes towards her since becoming an aphasic speaker. Her reflection of this (Box 1.4) includes concerns that professionals failed to see the extent of her personal loss. Her extensive abilities as a doctor with a very good education could be overlooked because of the way aphasia was interpreted by health professionals. It is too easy to use a benchmark of whether the individual can make basic requests and manage routine daily activities without due regard for the individual variations in how people live their lives. Those people who rely heavily on high-level language skills will face many challenges when coping with an acquired communication impairment because of the difficulties in accessing their premorbid status.

## Box 1.4 M's frustrations with the attitudes of others

'To be told I ought to be thankful that I'd got speech at whatever level ... I couldn't read philosophy ... I had before and I wanted to again ... I wanted to make sense out of it and in the early days it's so difficult. I think it was the fact that I was being patronised ... you know it puts you back very much to the childlike model where you feel like kicking their shin!'

'I was made to feel that I was being selfish in that I was wanting more, that I ought to be glad that I was as good as I was and that a lot of people were worse than that. And when I pointed out that a lot of people weren't as bright as me in the first instance it was when I got some really quizzical looks...why because you have had a medical catastrophe...why shouldn't you be striving to be what you were before? That is very patronising.'

'Most of us would settle for 75–80%, but so often the indication was well you've got 25% of what you were...think yourself lucky. One of the first times I actually found a torrent of words which was wonderful...didn't come out with a lot of sense but the feeling was when somebody told me I ought to consider myself 'lucky'. I started off swearing, which I didn't tend to do much before and asked her why she thought I was xxxxing well lucky when it was the most unlucky thing that ever happened. And she was shocked! Really quite badly shocked...well if it makes her think twice about saying the same to someone else...it's just as well.'

Help for coping with the effects will come from a variety of sources within the individual's own environment. In Box 1.5, M describes some examples of this, with evidence that friends in an entirely informal way, thought of ways to help. Professional contacts provided a different sort of support, and finally M developed solutions on her own through the walking and reliance on her own company.

### Box 1.5   M's sources of help and support

'A lot of the post operative care came from very good friends who encouraged me to do the quick crossword of the *Guardian* as therapy and now I usually miss about 2 clues whereas when I first started I would only get about 2 clues.'

'I've been very fortunate in that I had the support of colleagues and have had one catastrophe when I tried to do one workshop but for the last 2 years I've been president of a European Society and so have had to give presentations...so talk about having safety nets and backups...it's all written out, someone else can read it if I can't, I explain what's the problem at the start...so that I have the confidence to try and do it.'

'Basically it's the silent disability and nobody realises. On a bad day you go for a walk. You don't find people...you go and do something that doesn't need words...of any sort. I went for long walks. The dog has never been fitter!'

Factors which were recalled as helpful to her sense of well-being are reported in Box 1.6.

## Box 1.6 M's route to recovering her well-being

'I had some very good friends in the hypnosis society and they were doing some very good courses in neurolinguistic programming (a type of hypnosis) and that has been very helpful.'

*Interviewer: Can you say in any way how that did help you? What did it do?*

'It gave framework I think. I think that's where it helped most. The Speech and Language Therapist said that . . . when I'd been away for one of the weekends . . . it was almost as if I'd gone up a gear, I was finding words more easily, it was almost as if they were teaching me how to reopen blocked roads . . . certainly I feel that if you are looking at the metaphor of roads I feel I'm on the country lane rather than being able to go on the motorways.'

### Summary

M has built on her abilities throughout this long time of recovery and has created a successful professional life for herself in a different direction. She has been able to increase her knowledge and move forwards, working at international level in a branch of psychological medicine. However, in looking back at her experiences she reported that the support she gained from the healthcare system was limited, in her view. She has been struggling to cope with the loss of her significant skills as a doctor for a long time. M summarised her experience as: 'It's like trying to find your way in a cloud.'

### Acquired dysarthria

In looking at the impact of acquired dysarthria on the self concept, Walshe (2003) showed that for 31 participants, the dysarthria had a negative impact upon on the self concept and that this did not change over time. Unlike aphasia, acquired dysarthria represents a different challenge for the individual. For these people their reduced intelligibility may affect the success of their communication with others and they may face prejudice from listeners who perceive their speech as 'slow' or even as someone who is 'drunk'. Yorkston, Beukelman, Strand and Bell (2001) examined the subjective experiences of people with multiple sclerosis who have associated dysarthria. As part of the analysis of in-depth interviews, one of the emergent main themes was 'communicating is unpredictable'. Part of this theme referred to individuals' perceptions about being treated differently because of their speech. One participant recalled a difficult interaction with a store manager. She described the manager thus: 'she just looked like I was driving her nuts, like I was really frustrating her and bothering her' (Yorkston, Beukelman, Strand and Bell, 1999, p. 134). Over time these difficult experiences may influence how the individual develops an understanding of self and identity.

John is 75 years old and worked before retirement as a pharmacist. He had a left cerebrovascular accident (CVA) in 2003 and was left with significant difficulties with dysarthria. He was able to write about his experiences and these are presented below. In Box 1.7 he describes the early stages of his experience.

### Box 1.7    John recalls the immediate aftermath of his stroke

'I cannot remember much after this but I was told that I had suffered a mild stroke. I had another stroke a few days later and lost my ability to walk, swallow and speak. I was finally diagnosed with temporal arteritis and moved to another hospital. Thus began a five month period of tests, assessment and treatment of which I have very little memory. I can remember that I often felt marginalised and lonely when my wife wasn't there—most others didn't bother speaking to me when they realised that I couldn't carry on a conversation.'

'I accepted my lack of speech as part of my illness and thought that I would either die or be completely better in a short time.'

John has made useful observations of his communication successes and factors that affect the success, as recorded in Box 1.8.

### Box 1.8    John's observations on communication

'Older friends, probably because they cannot hear so well, often have difficulty with what I am saying whereas our young grandchildren, although they all live abroad and don't see us very often, can carry on a perfectly normal conversation with me—perhaps this is because they are competently bilingual although other young people also manage to understand me.'

'One thing that really annoys me is when someone pretends to understand what I am saying. I can tell immediately when that is the case.'

He was also able to reflect on his recovery, as he describes in Box 1.9.

## Box 1.9 John's first steps to recovery

'When I first started making sounds and began to speak again I thought I sounded stupid so I didn't say anything that wasn't absolutely necessary. Now I am getting more confidence and speak more but it sometimes tires me if I speak for a long time. I still find it hard to say certain words but when I get stuck I can use the sign alphabet with Julia but not many others know it. Otherwise I try another word or spell it out letter by letter.'

'My son made me a large board showing big letters of the alphabet and a few useful words which I could point to but using it was a slow process. Very gradually I became able to mouth odd words then make vague sounds of speech.'

'The gift of the ability to speak and be understood is taken for granted by almost everybody. It is only valued when it is taken away. Even a simple monosyllabic phrase like "Hi, how are you?" opens a new world of communication. It is a long hard road to recovery but it is well worth the effort in the end.'

## The experiences of being a carer

Although this book is focused almost exclusively on the patient experience, it is important to note the role of the carer, which will be critical to outcome. Often the experiences of people who care for individuals with acquired communication impairments are overlooked. Managing to care for an individual who has a significant acquired communication impairment as well as low mood associated with this, is extremely challenging. The carer, particularly if he or she is the spouse or long-term partner, may go through a period of shock and anxiety while waiting to see if the individual will survive the stroke or brain injury. Then they have to cope with the information that their partner may survive but with a substantial degree of disability. Healthcare services rely on carers having the personal capacity to provide this sort of support. However, the literature shows that this is not easy. Personal accounts of coping (Hale, 2002) report on the difficulties in adjusting to the disability and the strength needed to manage over time. Pound, Parr and Duchan (2001) interviewed four women whose husbands had aphasia and their views were analysed in order to develop professionals' understanding about how to develop the content of a support course for spouses in the same situation. The interviews revealed that there were individual differences between the four women in terms of how they responded to their husband's aphasia. A range of problems emerged across the four interviews, which focused on the main themes of:

- difficulties in coping with changed and difficult behaviours on the part of the husband;
- coping with the effects of a partnership that was premorbidly difficult;
- balancing the demands and needs of other family members;

- managing time to take care of self, domestic activities and work;
- dealing with other people's responses to the husband's aphasia;
- negative feelings of uncertainty and despair. (Pound, Parr and Duchan, 2001)

Professional healthcare services such as Clinical Psychology and Speech and Language Therapy have developed in a variety of settings in different countries and the approaches to interventions for well-being may vary. Attention to the individual and carers feelings and emotional well-being may be prioritised in some working contexts and less so in others. This may be because of attitudinal factors but may also be related to resourcing issues and the limited number of health professionals who work in this specialised area.

There are many associations that help people with acquired communication impairments and their families. Some of these are privately funded organisations, some are organised through the NHS, and some are set up by individuals with aphasia who run web pages and conferences to help support people with acquired communication impairments and their families. Connect, the communication disability network (www.ukconnect.org), has developed a wide range of innovative approaches to helping aphasic speakers and their families. The recent publication *Caring and Coping* (Connect, 2008) provides guidance for people with aphasia and their family and friends. The Nottingham Speech and Language Therapy Service runs a special clinic to help aphasic speakers and their families (see 'Beyond words—a counselling service for clients with communication disability'; http://www.tin.nhs.uk/events-calendar/inspiring-success-2006/finalists/counselling-service).

Also web pages set up by aphasic speakers are providing a lot of help for individuals and their families (Aphasia Now; http://www.aphasianow.org/) and have created opportunities for people to link together and gain support. Holland (2007) provides extensive advice to professionals about how to counsel people with acquired communication impairments, and the families of such people. The chapter on how to counsel families containing a patient with a progressive disease provides an excellent source for professionals.

Julia is John's wife. They met at university and she also worked as a pharmacist. She provided some comments on her experiences during John's illness and recovery. In Box 1.10 she describes her memory of the early stages.

**Box 1.10   Julia's reactions to her husband's stroke**

'When John had a stroke and was taken to hospital I was in a state of complete shock. Although he had not felt well for a few weeks he had covered it up and pretended it was nothing particularly serious.'

'We have no relatives in Britain but as soon as John was taken to hospital our daughter caught the first available flight from Cyprus and before she went back our son drove from Luxembourg. They and their families have been, and continue to be, a tremendous support to both John and me. Most days I speak to them on the phone to let them know how John is getting on.'

'When John was first in hospital his walking got worse, he started choking on food and after ten days, whilst having a short service with the hospital chaplain, his voice just faded away. He never made another sound for over three months; he couldn't mouth words, in fact he couldn't even move muscles to smile for a few weeks.'

Julia made a series of useful observations on her experience of John's communication, as recorded in Box 1.11.

### Box 1.11 Communicating with John — beginning again

'John gradually became more alert to his surroundings and started mouthing words. After three months in hospital, when I was leaving one evening, I bent over to kiss him and he whispered "Night, night". I was so excited I could have shouted the news from the rooftops. That was the beginning but he often couldn't make any noise at all although on other occasions he managed odd words in a gruff voice.'

'At first most of John's words were difficult to make out, which was very frustrating for both of us—for John that he could not make me understand and for me because I felt guilty that I couldn't understand and I really wanted to help him. Even now, if John suddenly changes the subject, I occasionally have difficulty in following what he is saying and have to enquire as to what we are talking about.'

Julia noted John's improvement and gave an example of how things had changed since the beginning of his illness, recounted in Box 1.12.

### Box 1.12 Perseverance and progress

'I don't like going out without John unless a friend can sit with him. Once, however, I had to pop out for about half an hour and leave John on his own so I left the phone at his side in case he needed to get in touch with me urgently. When I got back a friend had rung and John had answered the phone for the first time in four years. I was really thrilled to learn from the friend that she had been able to carry on a normal conversation with John and could understand everything he had said. I'm so proud of John for his perseverance and progress with his speech.'

Over time the views of people who live with someone who has an acquired communication impairment develop and mature, and here with Julia it is possible to see how her care and support for her husband has been a positive influence on how they have both coped.

## What do these personal views tell us?

Although the experiences of each person are different and reflect the variable ways the communication impairment has impacted on them, there are also some commonalities. The confusion and uncertainty at the time of the acute illness are common to all, along with the shared anxiety about the future. There is a shared desire to get better and to improve, which the communicatively impaired speakers quoted here refer to by using the image of a 'long hard road' and a 'country lane instead of a motorway'. This image of moving along some sort of route fits with the general health narrative of a recovery trajectory, where the individual experiences an acute illness and then struggles towards improvement. All three refer to the significant changes that have occurred: the loss of employment and professional role, the social limitations and the ways in which the individual has had to learn to cope in society. In order to avoid struggling with speech there is a tendency not to speak, or to give up when factors affect the capacity to understand such as effects background noise. There are the reported difficulties when trying to understand each other and the need to develop strategies to manage this. The difficulties in understanding are based not just on the communication of the message from one person to another, but in the way other people fail to understand the impact on the speaker of losing speech. Both speakers refer to annoyance and even anger when people pretend to understand them, or at worst make assumptions about how they should be feeling ('I think it was the fact that I was being patronised'). There is positive recognition of change and improvement, as marked by success in speech being understood by a listener, or achieving the level of giving a public presentation, or being able to leave John and let him answer the telephone successfully. There is, finally, a shared complexity of experience: the communication impairment seeps into all aspects of individuals' lives ands shapes their future.

## Conclusion

This introductory discussion has aimed to highlight the key aspects of the conditions, along with examples of personal experience and discussion of important factors.

One of the most important aspects to emerge from this chapter is the complexity of the conditions described. When there is a communication impairment along with a physical condition a huge range of factors become relevant and important to clinical management. Inevitably this means that the assessment of the condition and decisions about intervention will involve a variety of health professionals. The benefit from this is that the patient is seen from a wide variety of perspectives, so that the sharing of knowledge between professionals will result in a better outcome for the patient. It is hoped that the considerations brought out in the introduction along with the detailed discussions in subsequent chapters provide a direction and focus for the health professionals of the future.

## References

Anderson G. Post stroke depression and pathological crying: clinical aspects and new pharmacological approaches. Aphasiology 1997;11:651–664.

Auerbach S, Kerow M. Neurobehavioural assessment of mood and affect in patients with neurological disorders. Semin Speech Lang 2003;24:131–143.

Brumfitt SM. A psychosocial case discussion. In: Proceedings from British Aphasia Conference, University of Cambridge, 1989; pp. 137–147.

Brumfitt SM, Sheeran P. VASES: Visual Analogue Self Esteem Scale. User's Manual. Oxon, UK: Winslow Press, 1999.

Bury M. The sociology of chronic illness: a review of research and prospects. Sociol Health Ill 1991;13:451–468.

Byng S, Kay J, Edmundson A, Scott C. Aphasia tests reconsidered. In: Code C, Muller D (eds) Forums in Clinical Aphasiology. London: Whurr, 1996; pp. 117–142.

Charmaz L. The body, identity and self: adapting to impairment. Sociol Quart 1995;36: 657–680.

Code C. The quantity of life for people with chronic aphasia. Neuropsychol Rehabil 2003;13:379–390.

Code C, Herrmann M. The relevance of emotional and psychosocial factors in aphasia to rehabilitation. Neuropsychol Rehabil 2003;13:109–132.

Communicating Quality 3. The Royal College of Speech and Language Therapists, 2006.

Collins English Dictionary. London and Glasgow: William Collins and Son, 1979.

Connect. Caring and Coping: a Guide for People with Aphasia, Their Family and Friends. London: Connect Press, 2008.

De Wit L, Putman K, Baert I, Lincoln NB, Angst F, Beyens H et al. Anxiety and depression in the first six months after stroke: a longitudinal multicentre study. Disabil Rehabil 2008;30:1858–66.

Duchan J, Byng S. Broadening the Discourse and Extending the Boundaries. Psychology Press, 2004.

Ellis AW, Young A. Human Cognitive Neuropsychology. London: Lawrence Erlbaum, 1988.

Faircloth CA, Boylstein C, Rittman M, Young ME, Gubrium J. Sudden illness and biographical flow in narratives of stroke recovery. Sociol Health Ill 2004;26:242–261.

France J. Disorders of communication and mental illness. In: France J, Kramer S (eds) Communication and Mental Illness: Theoretical and Practical Approaches. London: Jessica Kingsley, 2001; pp. 15–26.

Gainotti G. Emotional, psychological and psychosocial impairments of aphasic patients: an introduction. Aphasiology 1997;11:635–650.

Gravell R, France J (eds). Speech and Communication Problems in Psychiatry. London: Chapman & Hall, 1991.

Hale S. The Man who Lost his Language. London: Penguin Press. 2002.

Holland A. Counselling in Communication Disorders. Plural Publishing, 2007.

Howard D, Franklin S. Missing the Meaning? A Cognitive Neuropsychological Study of the Processing of Words by an Aphasic Patient. Cambridge, MA: MIT Press, 1988.

Jordan L, Kaiser W. Aphasia—a Social Approach. London: Chapman-Hall, 1996.

Kay J, Coltheart M, Lesser R. Psycholinguistics Assessment of Language Processing in Aphasia. Psychology Press, 1992.

Kolb B, Whishaw IQ. Fundamentals of Human Neuropsychology, 5th edn. New York: Worth, 2003.

Mackay R. 'Tell them who I was': the social construction of aphasia. Disabil Soc 2003;18: 811–826.

Mesulam MM. Primary progressive aphasia. Ann Neurol 2001;49:425–432.

Moss CS. Recovery with Aphasia: the Aftermath of my Stroke. Urbana, IL: University of Illinois Press, 1972.

Newborn B. Return to Ithica. Element Books, 1997.

Parr S. Living with Severe Aphasia: the Experience of Communication Impairment after Stroke. Joseph Rowntree Foundation, 2004.

Parr S, Byng S, Gilpin S, Ireland C. Talking About Aphasia. Buckingham: Open University Press, 1997.

Parr S, Duchan J, Pound C. Aphasia Inside Out: Reflections on Communication Disorders. Buckingham: Open University Press, 2004.

Patten J. Neurological Differential Diagnosis, 2nd edn. London: Springer, 1996.

Pound C, Parr S, Lindsay J, Woolf C. Beyond Aphasia: Therapies for Living with Communication Disability. Bicester: Winslow, 2000.

Pound C, Parr S, Duchan J. Using partners' autobiographical reports to develop, deliver and evaluate services in aphasia. Aphasiology 2001;15:477–493.

Royal College of Physicians of London. Concise Guide to Good Practice. National Guidelines No 4: Use of Antidepressant Medication in Adults Undergoing Recovery and Rehabilitation Following Acquired Brain Injury. London: Royal College of Physicians, 2005.

Royal College of Speech and Language Therapists. Clinical Guidelines. Bicester: Speechmark, 2005.

Shallice T. From Neuropsychology to Mental Structure. Cambridge: Cambridge University Press, 1988.

Tanner DC, Gerstenberger DL. The grief response in neuropathologies of speech and language. Aphasiology 1988;2:79–84.

van der Gaag A, Smith L, Davis S, Moss B, Cornelius V, Laing S, Mowles C. Therapy and support services for people with long term stroke and aphasia and their relatives; a long term follow up. Clin Rehabil 2005;19:372–380.

Walshe M. The impact of acquired neurological dysarthria on the speaker's self concept. J Clin Speech Lang Stud 2004;12/13:9–33.

Whitworth A, Webster J, Howard D. Assessment and intervention in aphasia. Hove, East Sussex: Psychology Press, 2005.

Yorkston KM, Beukelman DR, Strand EA, Bell KR. Management of Motor Speech Disorders in Children and Adults. Austin, TX: PRO-ED, Inc., 1999.

## Internet resources

Aphasia Now: http://www.aphasianow.org (accessed 30 March 2009).

Connect: http://www.ukconnect.org (accessed 30 March 2009).

Beyond words—a counselling service for clients with communication disability: http://www.tin.nhs.uk/events-calendar/inspiring-success-2006/finalists/counselling-service (30 March 2009).

# CHAPTER 2

# Evaluation of Anxiety and Depression in People with Acquired Communication Impairments

**Shirley A. Thomas**

## Introduction: emotional consequences of acquired communication impairments

Aphasia results in a range of psychosocial changes in professional, social, familial and psychological areas (Herrmann and Wallesch, 1989). Much of our happiness and sadness comes from interacting with people (Code, Hemsley and Herrmann, 1999), and the severity of aphasia impacts upon the time spent in social and community activity (Code, 2003). It is not surprising then that communication impairments have emotional consequences, including depression and anxiety. Kauhanen *et al.* (2000) reported that 70% of patients with aphasia had major or minor depression at 3 months after stroke, and 62% were depressed at 1 year. The presence (Åström, Adolfsson and Asplund, 1993) and severity (Thomas and Lincoln, 2008) of communication impairment have been found to be predictors of distress after stroke. Mood impairments need to be treated because depression is associated with poorer rehabilitation outcome (Herrmann *et al.*, 1998) and lower quality of life (Jaracz, Jaracz, Kozubski and Rybakowski, 2002). Therefore it is important that anxiety and depression are assessed in order to identify who may have mood impairments and where intervention is required. The purpose of this chapter is to provide a review of assessments for anxiety and depression suitable for people with acquired communication impairments.

A systematic review of studies that diagnosed depression after stroke found that 71% of the 129 studies reviewed reported some exclusion of people with aphasia (Townend, Brady and McLaughlan, 2007b). Less than half of the studies reported screening or assessing aphasia, and not all studies referred to whether people with aphasia were included or not. This makes reviewing the literature on assessments for depression and anxiety more challenging as there is limited literature available and few studies have focused exclusively on people with communication impairments.

In studies that have included people with aphasia some still excluded those who had moderate to severe comprehension impairments or global aphasia after stroke (Robinson, Starr, Kubos and Price, 1983) and traumatic brain injury (Jorge et al., 2004). Starkstein and Robinson (1988) noted that 'At the present time we do not see any way to make reliable and valid diagnoses of emotional disorders in patients with comprehension deficits and feel that these patients should be excluded from studies in which the patient's emotional state is an important variable' (p. 16). It is hoped to show in this chapter that assessments have been developed that are appropriate for assessing mood in people with communication impairments.

## Assessing anxiety and depression

Assessments for anxiety and depression are used for a number of purposes. Firstly they can be used to screen for mood impairments, that is, to identify people who may have anxiety or depression. Screening is carried out with a large number of people, for example for all patients on a rehabilitation ward, and identifies people in need of more detailed investigation of their mood. The recognition of anxiety and depression in people with acquired communication impairments is important to improve treatment and outcomes. In addition to screening, assessments can be used to diagnose mood disorder and classify people as having 'anxiety' or 'depression'. Assessments can also be important to determine the severity of mood impairments, monitor change over time and evaluate the effectiveness of interventions. The focus of this chapter are assessments for screening and measuring the severity of mood impairments.

There is a paradox of how to study emotional disorder when the basic method used to assess it (i.e. language) is impaired (Starkstein and Robinson, 1988). Acquired communication impairments can impact upon the assessment of mood in a number of ways. Self-report assessments of depression and anxiety require comprehension of instructions, statements or questions and so can be difficult for those with receptive language impairments. Patients with expressive language impairments, including an unreliable yes/no response, inability to give a complex answer or having word-finding difficulties, will have impairments in responding to questions.

Methods for *diagnosing* depression are language based and include interviews, self-administered questionnaires (written modality) or verbally administered assessments (spoken modality) (Townend, Brady and McLaughlan, 2007b). This presents obvious challenges when working with people who have communication impairments. Traditional methods of assessing mood may have to be adapted so they are suitable. However, methods for *screening* for anxiety or depression do not have to rely on intact language skills as they can include picture-based (visual analogue) measures for self-report of mood and questionnaires designed for completion by an observer, such as ward staff, carers or relatives.

In a systematic review of 60 studies that diagnosed depression after stroke and included people with aphasia, almost half (48%) of studies adapted the diagnostic method for participants with aphasia (Townend, Brady and McLaughlan, 2007b). Methods of adaptation most commonly included supplementing interviews using informants (relatives or staff), followed by clinical observation, modifying questions or response options, and visual analogue scales. Studies varied in the level of detail they provided on the methods used, which would make replication difficult. Some people with milder communication impairments may be able to complete self-report measures with assistance from the assessor, but the reliability of this depends on the assessor not making assumptions or offering answers to questions (Code and Herrmann, 2003). Using assistance from relatives and staff to assess patients with aphasia on the Montgomery–Asberg Depression Rating Scale (MADRS) (Montgomery and Åsberg, 1979) decreased validity (Laska *et al.*, 2007) and so this may not be appropriate if the measure is not designed to be completed in this way. Although efforts to assess mood in people with aphasia represent positive progress in this area, the reliability and validity of the amended methods is not usually established. Rather than adapting existing methods it may be more appropriate to develop assessments specifically for people with communication impairments to ensure they are suitable.

## Choosing an assessment

When selecting or evaluating an assessment of anxiety or depression there are two main factors to consider. Firstly, the psychometric properties of the assessment should be reviewed; this includes the reliability and validity of the scale and, where relevant, the accuracy of cut-off points for identifying mood impairments. Secondly, the practicalities of using a measure with people who have acquired communication impairments needs to be taken into account. An overview of these properties will be provided and relevant assessments will then be reviewed.

A valid measure 'is one which can measure whatever it is supposed to, and can achieve the purpose wanted' (Wade, 1992, p. 37). There are several facets of validity and the following are particularly relevant to assessments of anxiety and depression:

- Content validity—whether the items in a scale represent all aspects of the construct being assessed (e.g. does it cover all symptoms of depression?).
- Concurrent validity—the correlation between a new scale (e.g. a new measure of depression) and a criterion measure (e.g. an existing 'gold standard' measure of depression).

- Construct validity—assesses whether the results of a test fit with the theory on which the test is based. The test should be correlated with other measures of the same construct (convergent validity) and not correlate with unrelated variables (discriminant validity).

A reliable measure is one that 'consistently produces the same results, particularly when applied to the same subjects at different time periods when there is no evidence of change' (Bowling, 1997, p. 11). The different components of reliability include:

- Internal consistency—this evaluates the homogeneity of the scale by assessing whether the items in the scale are correlated with one another. This can be calculated using Cronbach's alpha (range 0–1), which should be above 0.70 (Nunnally, 1978).
- Test–retest reliability—the consistency of the measure when administered to the same people on two occasions. A mood assessment should be measuring a stable and consistent response.
- Inter-rater reliability—the agreement between two raters assessing the same individual. This is relevant if the assessor has to interpret or score responses.
- Sensitivity to change—the ability of a measure to detect change. This should be evaluated if the measure will be used to monitor changes in mood over time or assessing outcome following intervention for anxiety or depression.

Reliability and validity are not synonymous. The reliability and validity of an assessment should be evaluated in the patient group with which the assessment is to be used, as these properties do not necessarily generalise from one condition to another. It cannot be assumed that a measure shown to be reliable and valid in one patient group will also be reliable and valid when used with people who have a different condition. This is particularly important when a cut-off on a scale is required to screen for anxiety or depression. More detailed information on the properties of measures is available in other sources (Wade, 1992; Streiner and Norman, 1995; Bowling, 1997).

As screening measures are used to identify people who may have a problem and require further assessment they will usually have a cut-off score such that a score above this point indicates the presence of a mood problem. When selecting or evaluating an assessment the accuracy of the cut-off value should be considered, in particular the sensitivity and the specificity. The *sensitivity* (true positive rate) of a test is how good it is at correctly identifying people who have the condition (e.g. correctly identifying people who are depressed as being depressed). The *specificity* (true negative rate) of a test is how accurate it is at correctly identifying people who do not have the condition (e.g. correctly identifying people who are not depressed as not being depressed). Sensitivity and specificity values can range from 0 to 1 (or can be reported as a percentage). Screening instruments need to have good sensitivity (>0.8) and also high specificity (>0.6) (Bennett and Lincoln, 2006). For screening measures the priority should be to minimise false negatives (high sensitivity and high negative predictive value) as it is important not to miss someone who may have mood impairments (Watkins *et al.*, 2007)

In addition to the psychometric properties of reliability and validity, there are also a number of practical considerations when choosing an assessment of anxiety or depression for use with people who have acquired communication impairments.

- *Practical considerations*—screening measures should be short and simple to administer (Bennett and Lincoln, 2006) as they are to be used with a large number of people. Patients who are depressed may have low motivation and could decline to complete lengthy assessments (Schramke *et al.*, 1998). Assessments to be used in an acute hospital setting also need to be suitable for administration at a bedside, avoiding the need for complex stimuli or materials. In a rehabilitation or community setting assessments can often afford to be more detailed.
- *Patient characteristics*—patients with acquired communication impairments may also have cognitive impairments, such as visual neglect and difficulties with memory, attention and concentration, which mean that the cognitive demands of an assessment must be considered. In cases where an assessment requires the patient to point at a stimulus or response, administration may need to accommodate physical disabilities such as hemiparesis.
- *Administration*—a range of professionals may be involved in mood assessment, including psychologists, nurses, doctors, and speech and language therapists. In services where this is the case the measure should not require specialist training and should be appropriate for use by clinicians from different disciplines.
- *Scoring*—the ease of scoring a person's responses and interpreting scores should be taken into account. Scoring instructions should be clear and unambiguous. Also, where information needs to be communicated to staff within a multidisciplinary team it is important that scoring can be easily explained and interpreted by other staff who may not be familiar with the assessment.
- *Cost*—the initial cost of purchasing the manual and stimuli for an assessment can influence whether it is adopted by a service, particularly where multiple copies are required. For some assessments there is the additional cost of purchasing individual response sheets/booklets. However, not all measures need to be purchased as some are freely available as appendices in published papers or from the scale's authors.

## Review of assessments for anxiety and depression

A wide range of assessments are available to assess mood in people with physical illness or disability who do not have communication impairments. These include, but are not limited to, the Beck Depression Inventory (BDI; Beck and Steer, 1987), Beck Depression Inventory II (BDI-II; Beck, Steer and Brown, 1996), Beck Depression Inventory FastScreen (Beck, Steer and Brown, 2000), General Health Questionnaire (GHQ; Goldberg and Williams, 1988), Hospital Anxiety and Depression Scale (HADS; Zigmond and Snaith, 1983) and the Beck Anxiety Inventory (BAI; Beck and Steer, 1993). Self-report questionnaires have been found to be sensitive but not specific for detecting depression in stroke patients without communication impairments (Lincoln *et al.*, 2003) and may be assessing distress rather than identifying depression and anxiety (Schramke *et al.*, 1998). There is no 'gold standard' method for diagnosing depression in aphasia and therefore no agreed standard to test screening measures against (Townend, Brady and McLaughlan, 2007a).

Existing self-report questionnaires can sometimes be used with people who have mild communication impairments, but they are not appropriate for people with moderate or severe communication difficulties due to the level of receptive and expressive language abilities needed to complete them. As a result, measures have been developed to assess mood in people with acquired communication impairments and these will be reviewed.

The simplest tool that has been used to screen for depression in stroke patients is the single-item Yale question 'Do you often feel sad or depressed? (Yes/No) (Mahoney and Drinka, 1994). In a sample of stroke patients the question had high sensitivity and specificity (>0.8) at identifying depression on the MADRS (Watkins *et al.*, 2007). Such a brief measure requires minimal training and could be used to identify those who require further assessment, but it has not been evaluated in people with severe communication impairments. The question requires a reliable yes/no response. Also, a single item with a dichotomous response does not provide information on severity, which would be used when evaluating response to treatment (Turner-Stokes, Kalmus, Hirani and Clegg, 2005).

### Self-report measures

Self-report visual analogue scales have been described as a valuable tool for assessing mood (Ahearn, 1997) and have been used to reduce the cognitive and linguistic demands on the respondent (Stern, 1997). Visual analogue scales originally consisted of an anchor word at each end of a 10-cm horizontal or vertical line, with the respondent putting a mark on the line to indicate the extent of endorsement. More recent versions have included simple pictures, such as happy and sad faces (Lee, Tang, Yu and Cheung, 2008), to illustrate the mood symptom asked about.

The ability of stroke patients to successfully complete visual analogue scales has been questioned. A study of inpatients within the first 6 months following a stroke assessed the ability to complete five types of visual analogue scale to rate the tightness of a sphygmomanometer cuff (Price, Curless and Rodgers, 1999). The stroke sample was less likely to correctly complete the scales than age-matched controls, although aphasia was not associated with mistakes at completing scales. Also, the scales included single words, numerical ratings and a vertical or horizontal line, and did not include pictorial representation, which may have assisted people with aphasia.

Although visual analogue scales allow a non-verbal response format the instructions are verbal (Townend *et al.*, 2007b). They are also limited in the range of symptoms they can depict (Herrmann and Wallesch, 1993). However, when self-report questionnaires are not appropriate, picture-based measures are a suitable method to collect information about someone's mood. Turner-Stokes and Rusconi (2003) suggest that pre-assessment of the ability to answer verbal and visual analogue type questions can inform the format of presentation to be used. Concomitant visuo-spatial difficulties may influence the choice of measure. Vertical rather than horizontal scales have been recommended (Price, Curless and Rodgers, 1999), as people with left-sided neglect may have difficulty using a scale presented horizontally.

### Visual Analog Mood Scales (VAMS) (Stern, 1997)

The VAMS were developed for use with neurological patients who may be unable to complete verbal mood measures due to communication or cognitive impairments. The scales include eight unipolar mood items: Afraid, Confused, Sad, Angry, Energetic, Tired, Happy and Tense. Each stimulus is presented on a separate page and consists of a 'Neutral' cartoon face and verbal label at the top of a 100-mm vertical line, with the mood face and corresponding label at the bottom of the line. The patient marks on the line to indicate how they are currently feeling. Items are scored by measuring from the Neutral end to the patient's mark, giving a score between 0 (lack of endorsement) and 100 (extreme endorsement of the mood state). The first page of the response booklet includes instructions and an example to go through with the patient. Detailed administration and scoring guidelines are included in the manual. The raw scores can be converted to T-scores using tables in the manual. A T-score has a mean of 50 and a standard deviation of 10 such that a T-score >50 shows that the individual scored above the mean of the standardisation sample. Items can be summed to give a total score of 0 to 800, with scoring reversed for the Happy and Energetic items. A raw score of $\geq 50$ on the Sad scale suggests that further assessment of mood state is required (Stern, 1997).

Normative data are available for healthy adults, psychiatric patients and older adults (Nyenhuis *et al.*, 1997; Stern, 1997). The VAMS correlated with other self-report mood measures in an adult sample (Nyenhuis *et al.*, 1997) and stroke patients (Arruda, Stern and Somerville, 1999;

Bennett *et al.*, 2006). In a sample of 100 stroke inpatients the internal consistency of the VAMS total score increased from 0.71 to 0.81 when the Happy and Energetic items were removed (Bennett *et al.*, 2006). The optimum cut-off for the total score was ≥224 (sensitivity 0.81, specificity 0.51) and for the Sad item was ≥23 (sensitivity 0.88, specificity 0.62) in relation to depression on the HADS (Bennett *et al.*, 2006), although patients with aphasia severe enough to be unable to complete the HADS were excluded. Chapter 6 contains further discussion of the VAMS.

### Visual Analogue Self-Esteem Scale (VASES) (Brumfitt and Sheeran, 1999a, 1999b)

The VASES was developed in response to language-based self-report measures, which are often unsuitable for people with acquired communication impairments. The scale contains 10 items, each stimulus card showing a pair of line drawings representing bipolar constructs (e.g. Cheerful/Not Cheerful) and a verbal label above each picture. The response scale is the same for each item and shown below each picture: ++ 'Very true of me', + 'True of me', and a neutral '0' between the two pictures. The scale includes a practice item of Depressed/Not depressed. Items are scored 1 to 5 and summed to give a total score of 10 to 50, with a higher score corresponding to higher self-esteem. Concurrent validity with the Rosenberg Self-Esteem Scale has been demonstrated (Brumfitt and Sheeran, 1999a; Vickery, Sepehri and Evans, 2008). Scores on the VASES have been found to be significantly lower in stroke inpatients compared with age-matched controls (Brumfitt and Sheeran, 1999a; Vickery, Sepehri and Evans, 2008). Although developed as a measure of self-esteem, the VASES is included in this review as evidence suggests it may be useful to assess mood. In a sample of 100 stroke inpatients, including people with communication impairments, the internal consistency of the scale was high (0.83), and increased (0.85) when the 'depression' item was included in the total score (Bennett *et al.*, 2006). The VASES was also significantly correlated with the anxiety, depression and total scores on the HADS, suggesting that the VASES (including the depression items) could be used as an assessment of mood. Appropriate cut-off values for the VASES to identify depression or anxiety have not been found, although the scale was not originally developed for this purpose. Patients with severe language impairment consistently endorsed items in the positive range of scores compared to patients with less severe language impairment and it was suggested that they may not have understood the task (Vickery, 2006).

Although the VASES may not be recommended as a screening measure because there are no published cut-offs, it could be used for monitoring mood over time and evaluating interventions (Bennett *et al.*, 2006) and also to indicate severity. The horizontal format may be questioned for use with people who have visual neglect. However, the VASES was found to be unaffected by visual acuity, memory or attention and was minimally affected by visuo-spatial impairment (Vickery, 2006). The VASES has been used in several stroke studies (Bakheit, Barrett and Wood, 2004; Vickery, 2006; Thomas and Lincoln, 2008; Vickery, Sepehri and Evans, 2008; Vickery *et al.*, 2008). Further discussion on the VASES is found in Chapter 4.

### Depression Intensity Scale Circles (DISCs) (Turner-Stokes, Kalmus, Hirani and Clegg, 2005)

The DISCs is a simplified single-item visual analogue scale designed to provide a graded assessment of depressed mood, particularly for those who have communication and cognitive impairments following brain injury (Turner-Stokes, Kalmus, Hirani and Clegg, 2005) (Figure 2.1). The DISCs is a six-point scale presented vertically. The stimulus is six circles of the same size with the proportion of the circle shaded grey increasing as you move from the bottom to the top circle. The bottom circle ('No depression', scored as 0) is white and the top circle ('Most severe depression', scored as 5) is shaded grey. The individual is asked to indicate which circle shows how depressed they feel that day. Responses are scored from 0 to 5. The DISCs was evaluated in a sample of 114 younger adults with complex disabilities caused by acquired brain injury (Turner-Stokes, Kalmus, Hirani and Clegg, 2005). Scores on the DISCs correlated significantly with the Beck Depression Inventory-II, Numbered Graphic Rating Scale (NGRS) and *DSM-IV* (*Diagnostic and Statistical Manual of Mental Disorders IV*) and had excellent test–retest reliability over a 24-hour interval. A cut-off of $\geq 2$ on the DISCs had sensitivity of 0.60 and specificity 0.87 at identifying a *DSM-IV* diagnosis of depression.

The DISCs is short and simple, which makes it appropriate for use in an inpatient setting. The authors of the scale provide administration in the original article and importantly note that the precise method of administration is adapted according to the communication and cognitive abilities of the individual. The DISCs may be promising as a brief screening scale for people who have acquired communication impairments. The scale does not provide detailed information but could be used to identify those in need of further assessment. Participants in the validation study had to have sufficient communication ability to complete the BDI-II and NGRS and be given a *DSM-IV* classification, and so evaluation is required in people with more severe communication impairments. The scale is freely available from the authors.

### Brief Assessment Schedule Depression Cards (BASDEC) (Adshead, Cody and Pitt, 1992)

The BASDEC was developed to assess mood in older adults in a hospital setting. It consists of 19 cards each presenting a statement derived from the Brief Assessment Schedule, for example, 'I've given up hope'. Each card is presented one at a time, and the respondent places the statement card next to a 'True' or 'False' card to indicate how they are currently feeling. True responses score 1 (except two items, which are scored 2), False responses score 0, and 'Don't know' scores 0.5, giving a total score between 0 and 21. Patients do not need to give a verbal response as they can place the statement card next to the True or False card. High sensitivity

**The Depression Intensity Scale Circles (DISCs)**

The DISCs is reproduced from the original with copyright permission from Professor Lynne Turner-Stokes, Northwick Park Hospital, Middlesex, UK

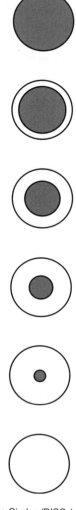

**Figure 2.1** The Depression Intensity Scale Circles (DISCs).

**Instructions for administration:**

**Say to the patient:**

This is a scale to measure depression

Please point to each of the circles in turn to make sure that
you can see them all.
[Continue only if satisfactorily accomplished]

The grey circles show how depressed you feel.

(Indicate the clear circle at the bottom)
The bottom circle shows no depression.

(Indicate the fully shaded circle at the top)
The top circle shows depression as bad as it can be.

(Pointing at each circle in ascending order)
As you go from the bottom circle to the top, you can
see that depression is becoming more and more severe.
Which of these circles shows how depressed you feel
today?

**To the administrator:**
In your opinion was the person able to understand this scale?

Yes.....
No.....

**Comment**

**Figure 2.1** *Continued.*

and specificity were found when the BASDEC was evaluated in elderly
medical patients (Adshead, Cody and Pitt, 1992; Loke, Nicklason and
Burvill, 1996). In a sample of 49 stroke patients (over 65 years old) a cut-off
of $\geq 7$ on the BASDEC had excellent sensitivity (1.0) and specificity (0.95)
at detecting *DSM-IV* major depression, and scores correlated with the BDI
FastScreen and HADS (Healey, Kneebone, Carroll and Anderson, 2008).
However, patients with severe communication impairment were excluded
if they were unable to complete the depression scales and interview.

The administration format of the BASDEC is appropriate for people
with acquired communication impairments, particularly in a hospital
environment, as each statement is presented individually and response
options are consistent. It does require people to be able to read the
statement or understand the verbal reading of items, and so may not
be suitable for those with moderate or severe receptive communication
impairments. The BASDEC may be appropriate for people with expressive

aphasia but good comprehension as verbal responses can be substituted by putting cards in the appropriate true/false pile, but further research with this group is needed (Healey, Kneebone, Carroll and Anderson, 2008). The BASDEC cards have to be purchased.

## Observer-rated measures

In addition to self-report methods, measures have been developed that are designed for completion by an observer, such as a nurse, carer or relative. Nurses have frequent contact with patients and so can have an active role in identifying depression (Klinedinst, Clark, Blanton and Wolf, 2007; Lightbody *et al.*, 2007b). The validity of asking informants to rate subjective cognitive symptoms of depression (e.g. worthlessness) is questioned (Townend, Brady and McLaughlan, 2007b) but observers can provide information about behavioural symptoms of mood impairments, such as weeping spells, taking an interest in activities, and sleep and appetite changes. This may be helpful when limited information can be gathered from self-report. However, the reliance on vegetative symptoms may also be criticised because people who have had a brain injury may present with symptoms such as sleep and appetite disturbances for reasons other than low mood (Starkstein and Robinson, 1988), such as hospitalisation and effects of the illness.

Family caregivers of people who have had a stroke have been found to have greater agreements with patient self-report when few depressive symptoms were present, while congruence between reports was lower when carers themselves reported fewer depression symptoms (Klinedinst, Clark, Blanton and Wolf, 2007; Townend, Brady and McLaughlan, 2007a). Therefore it is important to take into account the mood of a carer when asking them to evaluate a patient's mood.

## Signs of Depression Scale (SODS) (Hammond, O'Keefe and Barer, 2000)

The SODS was developed as a depression screening tool to be completed by an observer, such as a nurse. The six items for the scale were identified from observable behaviours in *DSM-III-R* (*Diagnostic and Statistical Manual of Mental Disorders III Revised*) criteria for depression and symptoms found to discriminate depression in those with physical illness. The items ask about the patient looking sad, crying, agitation or restlessness, needing encouragement to do things and seeming withdrawn. Answers to each question are yes/no to avoid ambiguity. Items are scored as 0 (No) or 1 (Yes) and summed to give a total score of 0 to 6. The original questionnaire was validated on a sample of patients on acute geriatric wards. The SODS has been evaluated with stroke patients (Watkins *et al.*, 2001; Bennett *et al.*, 2006; Lightbody *et al.*, 2007a). Scores correlated with the HADS depression and total scores but the internal consistency at 0.53 was low

(Bennett *et al.*, 2006). The recommended cut-off of ≥2 had sensitivity of 0.64 and specificity 0.61 at identifying a clinical diagnosis of depression from a psychiatrist in a sample of stroke inpatients (Lightbody *et al.*, 2007a). The optimum cut-off was the same when the subgroup of patients with communication impairments was examined separately. The optimum cut-off when carers completed the scale was higher at ≥4, and agreement between nurses and carers was only fair (Lightbody *et al.*, 2007a).

The SODS is quick to complete and so is appropriate for use in a hospital setting to identify people whose mood should be monitored or assessed in more detail. It is commendable that the scale has been evaluated against a psychiatrist's diagnosis of depression in a sample that included people with communication impairments. The scale is also acceptable for use with carers, who may be able to assist in identifying behavioural symptoms of depression, although in carers of people who had multiple sclerosis, the carers' mood was correlated with SODS scores (Groom, Lincoln, Francis and Stephan, 2003). The sensitivity and specificity of the cut-off value are below the recommended levels for a screening measure and so people with depression may be missed. Respondents may find it difficult to classify some answers as yes or no, and this also loses detail about gradual changes for an item. The items for the SODS are reported in the original publication of the scale (Hammond, O'Keefe and Barer, 2000).

### Stroke Aphasic Depression Questionnaire (SADQ) (Sutcliffe and Lincoln, 1998) and Hospital Stroke Aphasic Depression Questionnaire (SADQ-H) (Lincoln, Sutcliffe and Unsworth, 2000)

The SADQ was developed to assess behaviours associated with depression in people with aphasia. The items for the scale were derived from existing depression questionnaires. The questionnaire is completed by a nurse or carer. Both the SADQ and SADQ-H have the same 21 items, for example, 'Did he/she have weeping spells?', and assess the frequency of the behaviour over the past week. The response options for the SADQ are Often, Sometimes, Rarely, Never. For the SADQ-H the response items were reworded to Every day this week, On 4–6 days this week, On 1–4 days this week, Not at all this week, as hospital staff completing the original version found the response options to be vague (Lincoln, Sutcliffe and Unsworth, 2000). Items are scored from 0 to 3, with a higher score indicating low mood, and are summed giving a total of 0 to 63. There are shorter 10-item versions of both the SADQ (Sutcliffe and Lincoln, 1998) (Figure 2.2) and SADQ-H (Bennett *et al.*, 2006), which give a total score of 0 to 30.

For the SADQ10 the optimum cut-off was ≥15, which had a sensitivity of 0.70 and a specificity of 0.77 for detecting depression on the Geriatric Depression Scale on a stroke rehabilitation unit (Leeds, Meera and Hobson, 2004). A cut-off of ≥18 on the SADQ-H had high sensitivity (1.0) and specificity (0.81), and a cut-off of ≥6 on the SADQ-H10 also had high sensitivity (1.0) and specificity (0.78) at identifying depression using the HADS

Please indicate how often in the last week the patient has shown the following behaviours:

1. **Does he/she have weeping spells?**

    Often          Sometimes          Rarely          Never

2. **Does he/she have restless disturbed nights?**

    Often          Sometimes          Rarely          Never

3. **Does he/she avoid eye contact when you talk to him/her?**

    Often          Sometimes          Rarely          Never

4. **Does he/she burst into tears?**

    Often          Sometimes          Rarely          Never

5. **Does he/she indicate suffering from aches and pains?**

    Often          Sometimes          Rarely          Never

6. **Does he/she get angry?**

    Often          Sometimes          Rarely          Never

7. **Does he/she refuse to participate in social activities?**

    Often          Sometimes          Rarely          Never

8. **Is he/she restless and fidgety?**

    Often          Sometimes          Rarely          Never

9. **Does he/she sit without doing anything?**

    Often          Sometimes          Rarely          Never

10. **Does he/she keep him/herself occupied during the day?**

    Often          Sometimes          Rarely          Never

**Figure 2.2** Stroke Aphasic Depression Questionnaire 10 (SADQ10). Sutcliffe, LM, Lincoln, NB, 1998. The Assessment of Depression in Stroke Patients: The Development of the Stroke Aphasic Depression Questionnaire. *Clin Rehab* **12**: 506–513. Reprinted with permission from Sage Publications.

(Bennett *et al.*, 2006). The SADQ-H and SADQ-H10 correlated with the HADS, suggesting the scale has concurrent validity as a measure of mood.

The SADQ is easy to use for untrained staff (Sackley, Hoppitt and Cardoso, 2006) and was specifically developed for stroke patients with aphasia. There are hospital and community versions, and the shorter 10-item version may be preferred in a setting where a briefer measure is required. The SADQ-H and SADQ-H10 were correlated with the total score on the HADS, and so may also assess overall distress. The SADQ and SADQ-H have been evaluated against self-report depression measures rather than a psychiatric interview for depression diagnosis. Studies have excluded patients with moderate or severe communication impairments as they were unable to complete the reference depression measures. The sensitivity of the scale to detect change in mood over time or following intervention has not been investigated. Future studies are required to evaluate the SADQ in patients who have severe communication impairments and are unable to complete self-report measures (Salter *et al.*, 2007). The versions of the SADQ are available from the published papers on the scale.

### Post-Stroke Depression Rating Scale (PSDRS) (Gainotti *et al.*, 1997)

The PSDRS is a 10-item observer-rated scale to assess depression in people who have had a stroke. The 10 sections are completed following an interview with the patient and cover depressed mood, guilt feelings, thoughts of death and/or suicide, vegetative disorders, apathy and loss of interest, anxiety, catastrophic reactions, hyperemotionalism, anhedonia and diurnal mood variations. Each section is scored from 0 to 5 apart from anhedonia, where scores range from −2 to +2. Rather than giving a global score, the PSDRS provides a symptom profile. Patients with language disorders were excluded from the evaluation study if they could not complete the verbal interview (Gainotti *et al.*, 1997).

The strength of the PSDRS is that it was developed for stroke patients although it provides a profile rather than an overall score, which may limit its use. It is completed following an interview and so requires training to use and cannot be completed quickly with a large number of people. There is little published information on the PSDRS and further evidence of reliability and validity is required before it could be recommended for routine use.

### Aphasic Depression Rating Scale (ADRS) (Benaim, Cailly, Perennou and Pelissier, 2004)

The ADRS is a nine-item behavioural depression rating scale developed for stroke patients who have aphasia. The items were developed using behavioural items from existing depression scales and include: (1) insomnia, (2) anxiety-psychic, (3) anxiety-somatic, (4) somatic symptoms-gastrointestinal, (5) hypochondriasis, (6) loss of weight, (7) apparent sadness, (8) mimic-slowness of facial mobility (non-affected side) and (9) fatigability (taking into account any motor deficiency). The number and wording of the responses differ for each item and items are weighted. The validation study of stroke patients in the first 6 months after stroke included patients with aphasia. The ADRS correlated with Visual Analogue Scales and the Hamilton Depression Rating Scale (the latter was only completed with those who did not have severe aphasia), supporting the construct validity of the scale. Test–retest reliability over a 2-week period and inter-rater reliabilities were high (average 0.69). Using a cut-off of ≥9 out of 32, the ADRS had high sensitivity (0.83) and specificity (0.71) compared with a psychiatrist's diagnosis of depression.

The scale is short and the items were derived from existing validated depression scales. Reliability and validity was found to be good by the scale's authors. The ADRS is to be completed by a member of the rehabilitation team or a psychiatrist based on interview and/or observation and therefore requires training to administer. The large number of somatic items in the scale may lead to inflated scores (Salter *et al.*, 2007). Benaim, Cailly, Perennou and Pelissier (2004) noted that the ADRS is suitable for completion for all patients and suggested that the VAMS could be used as a self-report measure as part of the clinical evaluation of mood. Further independent evaluation of the scale is required in a sample including patients with a broad range of aphasia severity. The items for the scale are included in the appendix of the published paper.

## Conclusions

Communication impairment can be a challenge to assessing mood but this does not mean that you cannot assess mood in people with acquired communication impairments. This chapter has illustrated that appropriate methods are available. The assessments described have assessed low mood or depression. No measures were identified that specifically focused on anxiety; this reflects the fact that depression has received the most research attention. Most of the studies have been conducted with stroke and neurological patients. Further work is required to identify appropriate methods for assessing anxiety in people with communication impairments.

The two main methods reviewed were self-report measures and observer-rated measures, and a combination of these can be used to assess mood. Observer-rated measures have been developed that are completed by a member of staff, relative or carer (e.g. SADQ, SADQ-H and SODS). This means it is important to educate staff and family members about the emotional consequences of acquired communication impairments and recognising symptoms of anxiety and depression. Many symptoms of depression are subjective so assessment should still involve self-report (Townend, Brady and McLaughlan, 2007b). Visual analogue scales with a simple format (VAMS, VASES and DISCS) have been developed for evaluating self-reported mood in people with communication impairments. These measures still require verbal instructions, which need to be presented in a format appropriate for people with comprehension difficulties. Also, clinicians should receive training in supported communication to enable them to communicate appropriately with patients when completing assessments.

Patients vary in the profile of communication impairments they experience so there is not one particular assessment that can be applied to all patients and settings. As outlined in this chapter, assessments can be used for a number of purposes and there are a range of factors to consider when selecting which one to use. People with comprehension difficulties were often excluded from studies and further evaluation of the appropriateness of existing assessments with this group is needed.

## References

Adshead F, Cody DD, Pitt B. BASDEC: a novel screening instrument for depression in elderly medical inpatients. BMJ 1992;305:397.

Ahearn EP. The use of visual analogue scales in mood disorders: A critical review. J Psychiat Res 1997;31:569–579.

Arruda JE, Stern RA, Somerville JA. Measurement of mood states in stroke patients: Validation of the Visual Analog Mood Scales. Arch Phys Med Rehabil 1999;80:676–680.

Åström M, Adolfsson R, Asplund K. Major depression in stroke patients. A 3-year longitudinal study. Stroke 1993;24:976–982.

Bakheit AMO, Barrett L, Wood J. The relationship betwen the severity of post-stroke aphasia and state self-esteem. Aphasiology 2004;18:759–764.

Beck AT, Steer RA. Beck Depression Inventory Manual. San Antonio, TX: The Psychological Corporation, 1987.

Beck AT, Steer RA. Beck Anxiety Inventory Manual. San Antonio, TX: Psychological Corporation, 1993.

Beck AT, Steer RA, Brown GK. Beck Depression Inventory Manual, 2nd edn. San Antonio, TX: The Psychological Corporation, 1996.

Beck AT, Steer RA, Brown GK. BDI-FastScreen for Medical Patients Manual. The Psychological Corporation, 2000.

Benaim C, Cailly B, Perennou D, Pelissier J. Validation of the Aphasic Depression Rating Scale. Stroke 2004;35:1692–1696.

Bennett HE, Lincoln NB. Screening for mood disorders after stroke: a review of potential measures for routine screening. Int J Ther Rehabil 2006;13:401–406.

Bennett HE, Thomas SA, Austen R, Morris AMS, Lincoln NB. Validation of screening measures for assessing mood in stroke patients. Brit J Clin Psychol 2006;45:367–376.

Bowling A. Measuring Health. Buckingham: Open University Press, 1997.

Brumfitt S, Sheeran P. The development and validation of the Visual Analogue Self-Esteem Scale. Brit J Clin Psychol 1999a;38:387–400.

Brumfitt S, Sheeran P. VASES: Visual Analogue Self-Esteem Scale. Bicester: Winslow Press Ltd, 1999b.

Code C. The quantity of life for people with chronic aphasia. Neuropsychol Rehabil 2003;13:379–390.

Code C, Hemsley G, Herrmann M. The emotional impact of aphasia. Semin Speech Lang 1999;20:19–31.

Code C, Herrmann M. The relevance of emotional and psychosocial factors in aphasia to rehabilitation. Neuropsychol Rehabil 2003;13:109–132.

Gainotti G, Azzoni A, Razzano C, Lanzillotta M, Marra C. The Post-Stroke Depression Rating Scale: A test specifically devised to investigate affective disorders of stroke patients. J Clin Exp Neuropsychol 1997;19:340–356.

Goldberg D, Williams P. A User's Guide to the General Health Questionnaire. Windsor: Nfer-Nelson, 1988.

Groom MJ, Lincoln NB, Francis VM, Stephan TF. Assessing mood in patients with multiple sclerosis. Clin Rehabil 2003;17:847–857.

Hammond MF, O'Keefe ST, Barer DH. Development and validation of a brief observer-rated screening scale for depression in elderly medical patients. Age Ageing 2000;29:511–515.

Healey AK, Kneebone II, Carroll M, Anderson SJ. A preliminary investigation of the reliability and validity of the Brief Assessment Schedule Depression Cards and the Beck Depression Inventory-Fast Screen to screen for depression in older stroke survivors. Int J Geriatr Psych 2008;23:531–536.

Herrmann M, Wallesch C-W. Psychosocial changes and psychosocial adjustment with chronic and severe non-fluent aphasia. Aphasiology 1989;3:513–526.

Herrmann M, Wallesch C-W. Depressive changes in stroke patients. Disabil Rehabil 1993;15:55–66.

Herrmann N, Black SE, Lawrence J, Szekely C, Szalai JP. The Sunnybrook Stroke Study: A prospective study of depressive symptoms and functional outcome. Stroke 1998;29:618–624.

Jaracz K, Jaracz J, Kozubski W, Rybakowski JK. Post-stroke quality of life and depression. Acta Neuropsych Scand 2002;14:219–225.

Jorge RE, Robinson RG, Moser D, Tatteno A, Crespo-Facorro B. Major depression following traumatic brain injury. Arch Gen Psychiat 2004;61:42–50.

Kauhanen ML, Korpelainen JT, Hiltunen P, Määttä R, Mononen H, Brusin E, Sotaniemi KA, Myllylä VV. Aphasia, depression, and non-verbal cognitive impairment in ischaemic stroke. Cerebrovasc Dis 2000;10:455–461.

Klinedinst NJ, Clark PC, Blanton S, Wolf SL. Congruence of depressive symptom appraisal between persons with stroke and their caregivers. Rehabil Psychol 2007;52:215–225.

Laska AC, Martensson B, Kahan T, von Arbin M, Murray V. Recognition of depression in aphasic stroke patients. Cerebrovasc Dis 2007;24:74–79.

Lee ACK, Tang SW, Yu GKK, Cheung RTF. The smiley as a simple screening tool for depression after stroke: a preliminary study. Int J Nurs Stud 2008;45:1081–1089.

Leeds L, Meera RJ, Hobson JF. The utility of the Stroke Aphasia Depression Questionnaire in a stroke rehabilitiation unit. Clin Rehabil 2004;18:228–231.

Lightbody CE, Auton M, Baldwin R, Gibbon B, Hamer S, Leathley MJ, Sutton C, Watkins CL. The use of nurses'and carers' observations in the identification of poststroke depression. J Adv Nurs 2007a;60:595–604.

Lightbody CE, Baldwin R, Connolly M, Gibbon B, Jawaid N, Leathley M, Sutton C, Watkins CL. Can nurses help identify patients with depression following stroke? A pilot study using two methods of detection. J Adv Nurs 2007b;57:505–512.

Lincoln NB, Sutcliffe LM, Unsworth G. Validation of the Stroke Aphasic Depression Questionnaire (SADQ) for use with patients in hospital. Clin Neuropsychol Assess 2000;1:88–96.

Lincoln NB, Nicholl CR, Flannaghan T, Leonard M, Van der Gucht E. The validity of questionnaire measures for assessing depression after stroke. Clin Rehabil 2003;17:840–846.

Loke B, Nicklason F, Burvill P. Screening for depression: Clinical validation of geriatricians diagnosis, The Brief Assessment Schedule Depression Cards and the 5-item version of the Symptom Check List among non-demented geriatric inpatients. Int J Geriatr Psychiat 1996;11:461–465.

Mahoney JJ, Drinka TJK. Screening for depression: single question versus GDS. J Am Geriatr Soc 1994;9:1006–1008.

Montgomery SA, Åsberg M. A new depression scale designed to be sensitive to change. Brit J Psychiat 1979;134:382–389.

Nunnally JC. Psychometric Theory, 2nd edn. New York: McGraw-Hill, 1978.

Nyenhuis DL, Stern RA, Yamamoto C, Luchetta T, Arruda JE. Standardization and validation of the Visual Analog Mood Scales. Clin Neuropsychol 1997;11:407–415.

Price CIM, Curless RH, Rodgers H. Can stroke patients use visual analogue scales? Stroke 1999;30:1357–1361.

Robinson RG, Starr LB, Kubos KL, Price TR. A two-year longitudinal study of post-stroke mood disorders: Findings during the initial evaluation. Stroke 1983;14:736–741.

Sackley CM, Hoppitt TJ, Cardoso K. An investigation into the utility of the Stroke Aphasic Depression Questionnaire (SADQ) in care home settings. Clin Rehabil 2006;20:598–602.

Salter K, Bhogal SK, Foley N, Jutai J, Teasell R. The assessment of poststroke depression. Top Stroke Rehabil 2007;14:1–24.

Schramke CJ, Stowe RM, Ratcliff G, Goldstein G, Condray R. Poststroke depression and anxiety: Different assessment methods result in variations in incidence and severity estimates. J Clin Exp Neuropsychol 1998;20:723–737.

Starkstein SE, Robinson RG. Aphasia and depression. Aphasiology 1988;2:1–20.

Stern RA. Visual Analog Mood Scales Professional Manual. Odessa, FL: Psychological Assessment Resources Inc., 1997.

Streiner DL, Norman GR. Health Measurement Scales. A Practical Guide to their Development and Use, 2nd edn. Oxford: Oxford University Press, 1995.

Sutcliffe LM, Lincoln NB. The assessment of depression in aphasic stroke patients: the development of the Stroke Aphasic Depression Questionnaire. Clin Rehabil 1998;12:506–513.

Thomas SA, Lincoln NB. Predictors of emotional distress after stroke. Stroke 2008;39:1240–1245.

Townend E, Brady M, McLaughlan K. Exclusion and exclusion criteria for people with aphasia in studies of depression after stroke: a systematic review and future recommendations. Neuroepidemiology 2007a;29:1–17.

Townend E, Brady M, McLaughlan K. A systematic evaluation of the adaptation of depression diagnostic methods for stroke survivors who have aphasia. Stroke 2007b;38:3076–3083.

Turner-Stokes L, Rusconi S. Screening for ability to complete a questionnaire: a preliminary evaluation of the AbilityQ and ShoulderQ for assessing shoulder pain in stroke patients. Clin Rehabil 2003;17:150–157.

Turner-Stokes L, Kalmus M, Hirani D, Clegg F. The Depression Intensity Scale Circles (DISCS): a first evaluation of a simple assessment tool for depression in the context of brain injury. J Neurol Neurosurg Psychiat 2005;76:1273–1278.

Vickery CD. Assessment and correlates of self-esteem following stroke using a pictorial measure. Clin Rehabil 2006;20:1075–1084.

Vickery CD, Sepehri A, Evans CC. Self-esteem in an acute stroke rehabilitation sample: a control group comparison. Clin Rehabil 2008;22:179–187.

Vickery CD, Sherer M, Evans CC, Gontkovsky ST, Lee JE. The relationship between self-esteem and functional outcome in the acute stroke-rehabilitation setting. Rehabil Psychol 2008;53:101–109.

Wade DT. Measurement in Neurological Rehabilitation. New York: Oxford University Press, 1992.

Watkins C, Leathley M, Daniels L, Dickinson H, Lightbody CE, van den Broek M, Jack CIA. The signs of depression scale in stroke: how useful are nurses'observations? Clin Rehabil 2001;15:456.

Watkins CL, Lightbody CE, Sutton CJ, Holcroft L, Jack CIA, Dickinson HA, van den Broek M, Leathley MJ. Evaluation of a single-item screening tool for depression after stroke: a cohort study. Clin Rehabil 2007;21:846–852.

Zigmond AS, Snaith RP. The Hospital Anxiety and Depression Scale. Acta Psychiat Scand 1983;67:361–370.

# 3 Brain Injury and Psychological Well-Being

## Camilla Herbert

This chapter will briefly review the literature on the main problem areas following acquired brain injury (ABI) for the individual, including communication difficulties and the impact these can have on well-being and psychological adjustment. In addition the chapter will consider the impact of communication problems on the family system as this is such a crucial component of long-term support for people with brain injury. Assessment and treatment of psychological well-being after stroke is covered elsewhere in this book so this chapter will focus more on those aspects of assessment and intervention for psychological well-being that are relevant to communication problems arising from other forms of acquired brain injury.

## Acquired brain injury (ABI)

The term acquired brain injury (ABI) is defined here as an injury resulting from an external physical trauma to the brain (e.g. road traffic accident, assault), as well as brain damage secondary to tumour removal, viral infections such as encephalitis, meningitis and anoxia. Anoxia and hypoxia are often caused by heart attacks, respiratory failure, drops in blood pressure, and a low oxygen environment. If the blood flow is depleted of oxygen, irreversible brain injury from anoxia (no oxygen) or hypoxia (reduced oxygen) can result in just a few minutes. Subarachnoid haemorrhage is also often included within the term acquired brain injury. Although it has a vascular origin and is a form of cerebrovascular accident or stroke, these cases can often present with problems more similar to a traumatically injured client group than to those seen in a traditional stroke service.

Traumatic brain injury (TBI) occurs as a result of a physical trauma to the head. This can happen by:

- the stationary head being struck by a rapidly moving object (acceleration injury);
- the head moving fast and striking a stationary object (deceleration injury);
- penetrating head injury (e.g. a bullet wound);
- by rapid whiplash movements of the head.

Traumatic brain injuries as a result of road traffic accidents, and often falls, characteristically result in widespread diffuse axonal injuries, and a pattern of cognitive and emotional changes reflecting the particular vulnerability of the frontal and temporal lobes to acceleration/deceleration injuries. Assaults may result in more focal damage, i.e. more similar to stroke, but can be accompanied by additional emotional components depending on the nature of the assault, for example symptoms of post-traumatic stress disorder (PTSD).

Traumatic brain injury is predominantly a condition affecting younger people. More than two-thirds of those who sustain traumatic brain injury are under 30 years of age. The majority of traumatic brain injuries occur among people aged 15–24 years (Jennett and MacMillan, 1981). By comparison, half of all strokes occur in the over-75 age group. The ratio of male to female is between two and three to one for traumatic brain injury.

There are a number of useful categories in distinguishing the severity of traumatic brain injury. Each category is defined by length of time in coma and/or period of post-traumatic amnesia. The Glasgow Coma Scale is a numerical score given to head-injured patients, starting immediately after injury, to measure degree of unconsciousness. Post-traumatic amnesia is the length of time after injury during which the patient is unable to remember continuous events, even when the patient is apparently awake. Head injuries are classified as mild, moderate and severe:

- A *mild* head injury is defined as a person experiencing a brief loss of consciousness (i.e. less than 15 minutes), or who has not been unconscious at all, with a period of post-traumatic amnesia of less than 1 hour.
- A *moderate* head injury is defined as loss of consciousness of between 15 minutes and 6 hours, and a period of post-traumatic amnesia of up to 24 hours.
- A *severe* head injury is usually defined as being a condition where the patient has been in a coma for 6 hours or more, or suffers post-traumatic amnesia of 24 hours or more.

It is difficult to obtain precise data regarding the incidence of traumatic brain injury, due to variations in definition and methods of data collection. Jennett and MacMillan (1981) cited estimates of the incidence of hospitalisation following head injury in Great Britain and the USA as between 200 and 300 per 100 000 of the population. Head injury accounts for 10% of all Emergency Department attendances. Whilst most head injuries are minor, 10–15 per 100 000 population have a severe head injury per year, and 15–20 per 100 000 sustain a moderate head injury. Thornhill *et al.* (2000) reported high rates of moderate or severe disability at 1 year post-injury in a study of mild, moderate and severe head injuries (disability rates of 47%, 45% and 48% respectively) in Glasgow. For comparison, the incidence rate

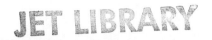

for stroke in the UK is 240 per 100 000, for subarachnoid haemorrhage (aneurysm) 10 per 100 000, and encephalitis 7.4 per 100 000 (Neurological Alliance, 2003).

## Impairments following acquired brain injury

Patients with acquired brain injury typically show long-lasting changes in cognitive, emotional and behavioural functioning. The nature and extent of the problems are related to the aetiology and severity of the damage, although patients with different aetiologies may show similar patterns of behavioural and emotional changes.

Improvements in acute care have resulted in reduced mortality rates in recent years. This, together with the relative youth particularly of those who sustain traumatic brain injury, has led to a rapid growth in the number of survivors of acquired brain injury living in the community. The vast majority of these survivors return to live with family members who are often ill equipped to respond to the changes in lifestyle and caregiver burden imposed by the injury and its cognitive, emotional and behavioural sequelae.

### Cognitive and communication changes

Traumatic brain injury commonly results in a pattern of cognitive problems secondary to frontal and temporal lobe damage, i.e. memory and dysexecutive problems. The damage can be global secondary to diffuse axonal injury or it can be focal. Aphasia and dysarthria do occur but many people with traumatic brain injury demonstrate intact speech ability. However, it is their poor conversational skills that can contribute directly to inappropriate behaviour in social situations and indirectly to the social isolation of themselves and their families. Talking too much, repeating the same topic or question, using inappropriate language for particular situations, or being unable to take turns in a conversation are all patterns of communication that affect people's ability to sustain relationships and/or return to employment.

### Emotional and behavioural changes

Traumatic brain injury often results in emotional and behavioural changes including emotional lability, impaired social perceptiveness, reduced self-control, and behavioural rigidity (Lezak, 1978; Bond, 1984). These deficits have a significant impact on the ability of these individuals to sustain employment, maintain close relationships, and participate in social and leisure activities within their community. Where there are communication difficulties all of these issues are magnified.

Depression, anxiety, fear and poor self-esteem are also common after brain injury. Emotional problems may be due to organic and non-organic causes, such as fear of what might happen, grief and anger about the loss of one's previous roles and status, panic because of the loss of control that comes with recognition of gaps in memory performance or inability to make oneself understood in public, and reduced self-esteem because of changes in physical appearance, verbal abilities, or involvement in the lives of significant others.

It can be difficult to distinguish between emotional and cognitive problems, and an interaction between the two may frequently occur, particularly where there is a lack of awareness in addition to the behavioural and personality changes. Communication impairments complicate this assessment still further.

## Psychological well-being

The incidence of psychological distress after acquired brain injury is generally high. The analysis is confounded by the problem of awareness, and the general pattern is that the more severely impaired, with lower levels of awareness, often show less depressed mood than those who are either moderately or mildly injured, where there is greater awareness of the changes in self and in role.

### Depression and suicide rates

Diagnosis of depression in both acquired brain injury and stroke populations is extremely problematic (Aben *et al.*, 2001; Evans and Levine, 2002). There is an overlap between somatic and cognitive symptoms of depression and the sequelae of acquired brain injury and stroke. Poor concentration, slowed motor and cognitive speed, fatigue and apathy, as well as problems with sleep, which are common manifestations of depression, are also frequently reported by non-depressed acquired brain injury patients. Nevertheless it does appear that depression rates after stroke and acquired brain injury are broadly similar, with around 20–40% affected at any point in time in the first year and about 50% of people experiencing depression at some stage.

The evidence suggests that the prevalence of depression within the traumatically brain-injured population increases with time after the first year post-injury. Traumatic brain injury leads to a particularly complicated form of psychological adjustment, with the varying levels of awareness, emotional denial, and the possible loss of the skills and opportunities to regroup and re-establish one's life. In addition these losses may be cumulative and ongoing such that a pervasive sense of grief may occur in the context of a disintegrated sense of self (Williams, Williams and Ghadiali, 1998). There is evidence of an increased suicide risk after traumatic brain injury of about three- or four-fold (Tate, 1997; Teasdale and Engberg, 2001; Fleminger, Oliver, Williams and Evans, 2003). Although some of this increased risk may be due to pre-injury factors in terms of the characteristics of people who suffer traumatic brain injury, increasing self-doubt and a sense of helplessness can cause the patient to withdraw, becoming more isolated and depressed. About 1% of people who have suffered traumatic brain injury will commit suicide over a 15-year follow-up.

### Rates of alcohol and drug use

Research indicates that pre-injury alcohol abuse was reported by as many as 79% of traumatically brain-injured people (Taylor, Kreutzer, Demm and Meade, 2003). A history of alcohol abuse was associated with lower levels of education, violence-related aetiology, and of being male, unmarried and unemployed. Pre-injury alcohol use is higher than in the general population. Pre-injury illicit drug use was described by up to 37% of the traumatically brain-injured people studied. Post-injury use of alcohol and drugs declines initially, but increases again as time elapses. The evidence suggests that patients who are less impaired are more likely to drink post-injury than more impaired patients. In some cases alcohol and drug abuse may become additional problems in an attempt to escape the inability to cope with the world (Sparadeo *et al.*, 1990).

## Why is acquired brain injury such a devastating psychological phenomenon?

As with brain damage secondary to stroke, there are three main factors causing the emotional and psychosocial disturbance after brain injury (Gainotti, 1993). First, neurological damage can affect the specific neural mechanisms subserving the regulation and control of emotional and social behaviour, resulting in a loss of emotional control and regulation. Second, psychological and psychodynamic factors involving attitudes towards disability and implications for quality of life affect how we think and respond, raising questions such as who we are as people, our self concepts, what roles we play, how we value ourselves and think we are valued by others. Third, there are the consequences of functional impairment on the individuals' social networks and social activities with their impact on family life and employment. Even a mild TBI can dramatically affect these factors, particularly the psychological and psychodynamic aspects. If, for example, your role at work is to be the person who chairs meetings, and generally acts as a resource for colleagues and staff, then even a mild slowing of information processing or a mild word-finding problem will reduce your effectiveness in the workplace, cause confusion in those who are used to depending on you, and potentially undermine your sense of who you are and how to function. To take on a different role, or a job with a lower status or less pay, may be a practical solution but it is not an emotional one. Social isolation is a major factor in terms of the impact of impairments on individuals and families. If you cannot return to work, a whole range of social contacts can be lost; if your partner cannot work because he or she becomes your carer, their social network tends to diminish; if your children do not feel able to bring home their friends because they are embarrassed by your speech or your behaviour then another opportunity for social contact is removed.

## Impact on the family

It is not just the person with the brain injury but also their family who is affected. There is an extensive literature on the impact of brain injury on family members (Perlesz, Kinsella and Crowe, 1999; Oddy and Herbert, 2003). Whilst studies of people with brain injury have often excluded people with communication impairments because of the difficulty of accurate self-report and engagement with the predominantly verbal measures of mood used, studies with relatives have been more inclusive, or at least less obviously exclusive of people with communication impairments

### Psychosocial burden on carers

In a series of longitudinal studies in the 1980s exploring family adaptation and distress, Livingston and Brooks (1988) described a pattern of rapidly developing high levels of distress over 3 months post-injury, which persist for 1, 5 and 7 years post-injury. Other authors have found similar raised levels of distress (Kreutzer, Gervasio and Camplair, 1994; Wallace *et al.*, 1998), and there have also been a number of studies reviewing family functioning and marital adjustment following traumatic brain injury that provide indirect evidence of stress and distress after brain injury (Moore, Stambrook, Peters and Lubusko, 1991; Douglas and Spellacy, 1996; Gosling and Oddy, 1999). Consistent relationships have been found between the relatives' perception as to the extent of the brain-injured person's deficits and in relation to particular changes in the brain-injured person. The level of stress experienced by the family is not clearly associated with the initial severity of injury in most studies (Oddy, Humphrey and Uttley, 1978; Brooks and McKinley, 1983; Gervasio and Kreutzer, 1997; Gillen, Tennen, Affleck and Steinpreis, 1998). A contrary finding is that of Douglas and Spellacy (1996), who found that 58% of variance in family functioning could be explained by severity of injury as measured by post-traumatic amnesia (PTA) in association with residual neurobehavioural function and adequacy of social support. In general it is the cognitive and personality changes that appear to be more related to family distress than any other consequences such as physical deficits or difficulties with activities of daily living (Oddy, 1995; Gosling and Oddy, 1999).

Many studies have concentrated on the first 2 years post-injury and show high levels of distress amongst family members in the immediate aftermath of the injury (Oddy, Humphrey and Uttley, 1978). Although some studies have not found a relationship between time since injury and stress levels in family members (Gervasio and Kreutzer, 1997; Gillen, Tennen, Affleck and Steinpreis, 1998), most studies that have followed families for 7 to 15 years have demonstrated that there are still high levels of distress and chronic strain in the families (Thomsen, 1984; Oddy *et al.*, 1985).

## Psychological assessment

As discussed previously, assessment of psychological distress in people with acquired communication problems is complex and dependent both on the level of communication impairment and on the usefulness of the available measures.

### Aphasia

Where an individual with an acquired brain injury has a primary aphasia the issues relating to the use of standardised questionnaires are similar to those for other groups of aphasic adults. For assessment after stroke Bennett *et al.* (2006) suggest as being appropriate for patients with communication problems the use of the Signs of Depression Scale (SODS) (Watkins *et al.*, 2001) in the acute phase, and the Stroke Aphasic Depression Questionnaire (SADQ) (Sutcliffe and Lincoln, 1998) or the Visual Analogue Mood Scale (VAMS) (Stern *et al.*, 1997) once people have moved into rehabilitation or into the community. Other authors have used the Depression Intensity Scale Circles (DISCs) (Turner-Stokes, Kalmus, Hirani and Clegg, 2005) or the Visual Analogue Self-Esteem Scale (VASES) (Brumfitt and Sheeran, 1999) (for further discussion on these assessments see Chapter 2). Where there are significant accompanying cognitive problems such as memory problems, it is important to recognise the need to focus the individual on their current mood state rather than expecting them to be able to reflect on mood over a day or week.

### Pragmatic skills

For many people with brain injury the communication impairments present as problems with social presentation. They show problems with word finding, excessive talkativeness, difficulty staying on topic, and poor turn-taking skills. As a result of their memory difficulties, slowed information processing speed or word retrieval difficulties they may have difficulty thinking of questions or comments to initiate or sustain a conversation, and struggle to keep up with a conversation in noisy environments or in a group. Problems recalling past and present conversation and events can limit the level of engagement in discussions and interactions. Difficulties in understanding more abstract language such as metaphor or sarcasm may mean that they present as humourless or 'missing the point' and at times this can result in misunderstandings, conflict and aggression.

Where an individual has fluent language skills but dysfunctional pragmatic skills that affect their social engagement and employability it can be helpful to use the La Trobe Communication Assessment (Douglas, O'Flaherty and Snow, 2000), which can identify where their higher level communication problems are having an impact on real-life situations. This can then form a basis for a therapeutic intervention, focusing on specific skills such as turn-taking and presentation skills, or on role plays for different social situations.

## Tangential speech and/or confabulation

This is an area where high-level communication impairment overlaps with cognitive dysfunction and/or mental health. Here verbal responses can be confabulatory or 'bizarre' and communication is affected. For example, Simon is a 24-year-old man whose right frontal lobe had to be removed after a block of wood fell on him in a work-related injury. Simon is otherwise physically fit but presents with lack of initiation, tangential speech and possibly with a mood disorder. However, any direct assessment or questioning produces tangential replies or questions in response. His responses to standardised language assessments are of questionable validity because Simon challenges individual items or gives bizarre and unscorable responses, and standardised assessments of mood or psychiatric disorder are similarly affected. Behavioural observation highlights concerns about self-neglect and withdrawal, which could be attributable to low mood, but can also be understood in terms of the impact of reduced initiation skills, i.e. as secondary to his brain injury rather than to a form of mental disorder or psychiatric diagnosis of depression. There is no evidence here of a formal language impairment; however, his tangential speech does result in a failure of communication ability.

One final area of communication impairment that has not been addressed is the impact of dysarthria, particularly at the higher level of functioning, where an individual is attempting to reintegrate into real-life environments and assumptions are made about them because of their speech. Kevin suffered a severe head injury and multiple orthopaedic injuries when he was knocked down by a car, and 8 years post-injury he is a 19-year-old man with an abnormal gait due to one leg being shorter than the other, dysarthric speech and cognitive impairment. Although his speech is mildly dysarthric he is normally fully comprehensible. However, in more stressful situations his speech becomes increasingly slurred and he can present as 'drunk', which causes him embarrassment both socially and in terms of interviews for work placements. Kevin is growing up as a young man with disabilities but with normal expectations of girlfriends, jobs and independence, and he is struggling to adjust to the gap between his aspirations and his opportunities. Although Kevin's other cognitive problems make it difficult for him to work at an abstract level in terms of psychosocial adjustment, he can work on goals that are directly relevant to things he sees as important.

He identified his slurred speech as an obstacle to his success in chatting up girls and was prepared therefore to work on a programme of anxiety management in social situations to address this. The programme involved identifying various elements in specific social interactions and practising conversation and options for dealing with them. Role play and video clips were used to provide additional material as Kevin had difficulty generating scenarios from his limited experience. By providing him with specific skills and opportunities to practise these in real-life settings, he was able to gain confidence in his ability to cope and he was able to succeed at interview and gain a part-time job in a local supermarket, where he interacted regularly with customers.

## Psychological interventions for well-being

### Direct interventions

### Cognitive behaviour therapy

Some patients can benefit from a cognitive behaviour approach to exploring their changed roles and sense of self, as this can provide the type of structure that supports impaired reasoning. Unfortunately the combination of communication and cognitive deficits often limits the patient's ability to deal with more abstract concepts, and poor memory skills may affect their ability to follow a discussion within a session or between sessions. Greater use of written or recorded material may be helpful, but less so for the more severely communication-impaired clients. The usefulness of metaphor and analogy can be limited, as rigid thinking and difficulty in generalising restrict the patient's ability to use these ways of thinking, but examples from day-to-day practice or from the patient's own experience can be used to build an account of incidents and social interactions that makes sense to that individual. Often the treatment needs to focus on addressing the limitations imposed by the injury, for example facilitating better access to enjoyable activities, rather than on the cognitions surrounding the changes in role and status.

### Psychotherapy

The sense of loss and the crisis of personal identity that often arise following brain injury raise questions for many patients such as 'Why did this happen to me?' and for some 'Is life worth living after this injury?' Patients who struggle with these questions also struggle to engage with neurorehabilitation and to identify achievable goals in their altered state (Prigatano, 1991). The anger and frustration that the first question engenders, and the depression and suicide risk that is often the consequence of the second question, are two reasons why some form of psychotherapeutic intervention is seen as desirable post-injury.

Nadell (1991) attempted to outline a psychological conceptualisation of what brain injury means to an individual. He focused on four central concerns of psychoexistential orientation: death, isolation, meaninglessness and freedom, and related these to the brain-injured experience. He argued that brain injury underscores our finite nature and imposes limitations in almost every sphere of existence from the basic functions (feeding, toileting) to the more complex activities of work, play and communication. Changes in cognition affect memory and symbolic thought, making the world a chaotic and confusing place from which the individual seeks to withdraw both physically and emotionally. Such a model sees the challenges confronting the brain-injured population as an intensification of the challenges confronting all human beings, and with the same requirements for specialised interventions.

The literature on the use of psychotherapy after brain injury focuses primarily on traumatic brain injury but also includes patients with the diagnosis of stroke, anoxia and other forms of acquired brain injury. In general the aetiology of the brain damage is not used as one of the criteria for determining appropriateness for psychotherapeutic intervention. It is the range and extent of the cognitive and awareness deficits that are most commonly referred to when discussing the use of psychotherapy, and in general communication-impaired patients are not routinely considered. The issues relating to insight and awareness are the primary focus of discussion, and assessing insight and awareness is particularly difficult where there are communication difficulties.

Unfortunately there is no obvious tool of measurement identified or criteria set that can be used to determine whether a client's cognitive or communication difficulties will affect engagement in psychotherapy. Bennett (1989), writing about patients with minor brain injury, included in his criteria for psychotherapy that 'the patient must demonstrate with reasonable probability the capacity to benefit, which requires the cognitive capacity to communicate his or her needs and to understand information communicated by the therapist'. Lewis (1991) also gave general guidelines for the success of psychotherapy with brain-injured patients, which include the requirement of the patient to have 'attributes and attitude conducive to the development of a sound working alliance'. Lewis did not argue that the patient has to be able to operate at a near normal cognitive level. She stated that initially the therapist and the environment must perform the functions of the lost areas—rather than functioning as the auxiliary ego as in supportive psychotherapy, the therapist is operating as auxiliary cortex, loaning intact cortical functions to the patient in order to offset the patient's experience of burden and deficiency. Similarly Ellis (1989) said that the therapist must be 'more active' than in traditional psychotherapy, using additional strategies to compensate for cognitive and personality changes.

Prigatano (1991) argued that the techniques used must 'make sense' to the patient as well as the therapist, and must take into consideration the cognitive and personality characteristics of the patient. He went further and stated that 'the psychotherapist of traumatic brain injury patients must demonstrate that the teaching methods are appropriate for a given patient and measure, directly or indirectly, the outcome of these interventions'. Building on case examples, he went on to say that 'the patients who seem to benefit most from psychotherapy are those who are committed to becoming independent, can take a realistic view of themselves, can see their strengths and weaknesses, and can work at cognitive remediation'.

## Behaviour management and training

Traditional behaviour management approaches did not address emotions but focused on changing behaviours, arguing that cognitions followed behaviours. By enabling people to 'behave' in a different way, it is possible to change how they 'feel'.

Anxiety disorders can emerge in relation to specific treatments or interventions and these can be addressed using a behavioural approach. The behavioural analysis may identify specific cognitive problems that are contributing to the individual's fear or anxiety in the situation, and the intervention may then consist of altering the way in which the treatment is delivered to avoid precipitating the fear or anxiety (Youngson and Alderman, 1992). Self-instructional techniques, particularly those based on repetitive practice, can help the patient to internalise the treatment approach. Although most studies have focused on patients without significant communication impairments, there is no reason why such techniques cannot be used for those with mild dysphasia. The concepts themselves are transferable, although the content of the repetitive practice may need to be modified. Malec (1994) describes a case in which a deficit of a patient's self-monitoring of her behaviour was thought to be contributing to her tendency to over generalise her assessment of negative events.

Social skills training is another area where behaviour analysis and role play have been important in helping patients to modify specific unhelpful behaviours and to acquire skills that develop new and more adaptive behaviours. This can be particularly useful around the pragmatics of communication.

## Family therapy

There are relatively few examples in the literature of family therapy in the traditional sense being used extensively with the acquired brain injury population, and particularly with those where communication skills form a significant part of the profile of impairments. However, many of the concepts and ideas that have evolved from the family therapy literature in terms of the dynamics within a family and the changing roles brought about by the trauma of the injury are increasingly being used to understand the emotional adjustment for individuals and their families (Perlesz, Furlong and McLachlan, 1989).

### Indirect interventions

### Environmental manipulation

This refers to managing the environment to provide positive experiences, sometimes working at the level of 'best interests' where the individual in question is extremely limited in their ability to communicate likes and dislikes, and interventions may be about identifying activities that provide pleasure (measured through observation of behaviour and responsiveness) and minimising those that are observed to produce a negative reaction.

### Education

This refers to the need to provide education to the individual, family, friends, staff and/or employers about the nature of the communication impairment and how to minimise its impact. This may involve a more family therapy type approach to help everyone in the family to understand where communication is failing, i.e. not just in terms of the individual with communication impairment, or it may be a more straightforward education session on what the individual can and cannot follow or say. Sometimes a single education session can be highly effective, and in other situations a more extended period of education and/or provision of written/visual information may be appropriate.

### Family training

In some cases it may be appropriate to engage members of the family network in managing an inappropriate communication style, both to help them cope and to give the individual concerned the best possible opportunities for social interaction, for example, providing direct feedback when certain topics are introduced, or by developing a system of gestures that highlight to the individual that they need to stop talking.

## Case studies

Case studies 3.1 to 3.3 illustrate different approaches to assessment and intervention for people with acquired brain injury.

---

### Case Study 3.1  Extremely severe impairment

Difficult and complicated questions can arise in relation to people with profound brain damage, where their ability to communicate is severely compromised. Assessment and interventions for psychological well-being are difficult but can be addressed. McMillan and Herbert (2000, 2004) report on a 5- and 10-year follow-up of the case of SG, and explored her mood and psychological adjustment. SG was severely brain damaged in a car accident and she was first assessed approximately 2 years post-injury (McMillan, 1996). At this stage SG's communicative ability was restricted to the use of a buzzer and/or finger movement, and it was unclear the extent to which her responses were purposeful. By the use of repeated presentation of counterbalanced sets of questions, and evaluating the consistency of her response it was possible to demonstrate that SG was responding consistently to simple questions relating to personal history but not to mood- or pain-related questions. Five years later (McMillan and Herbert, 2000) she was consistently able to give a verbal yes/no response to personal history questions and to closed questions about her mood/well-being, for example 'do you have pain in your leg?'; 'are you happy?'; 'do you like quiz games?' What she was not able to do at this time was to identify any activities or changes that could improve her situation if they were outside of her current daily experience. At 10 years post-injury (McMillan and Herbert, 2004) she was living with carers in her own adapted house and her quality of life was significantly enhanced as were her communication skills. She could give short verbal responses that were audible and comprehensible. She could interact with her carers, express preferences, and generally have a greater involvement in promoting her own well-being.

In another unpublished example, questions were asked about the psychological well-being of a 32-year-old woman who had been injured in a car accident 4 years previously. She was profoundly physically impaired and had no verbal language and limited attentional skills. Her husband was convinced that she understood everything that was said to her, that she was happy with the nature and type of personal care provided for her, and that she was able to participate in discussions concerning her care package. Staff at the nursing home had raised some questions about this, and sought advice as to her ability to engage in discussions.

Assessment, similar to that carried out with SG, identified that the patient could respond consistently with eye blinks only to basic biographical details (e.g. 'is your mother's name Sue?') but was unable to give consistent responses to questions in relation to presence or absence of pain, happiness/sadness or orientation to current environment. It was concluded that she was not able to direct her care package or to give guidance to the staff about her psychological well-being and factors that could affect it. The advice given to staff was to monitor her behaviours and responses to activities for signs of distress or pleasure and to use this to guide the care plan for her psychological health.

---

**Case Study 3.2 Severe expressive dysphasia**

*Brief history*
Peter is a 38-year-old man who suffered a severe head injury in a road traffic accident 2 years previously. His injury occurred when his car crashed into a tree, with no other vehicles involved. The full circumstances of the accident were not known. Although Peter had a history of excessive alcohol

consumption, there was no evidence of alcohol in his bloodstream at the time of injury. Two years post-injury Peter is a wheelchair user with limited functional use of his right side, but is independent, transferring with supervision only.

### Communication abilities

Peter is aphasic with no reliable verbal yes/no, and his gestures and minimal written prompts are of variable support in accurately conveying his meaning. The listener has to provide significant levels of support and interpretation even for basic conversational exchanges, and more complex discussions are of questionable validity. It is also unclear how well Peter retains information from session to session. There is evidence from functional activities that he needs repeated practice to grasp new techniques, and from discussions that he has either not fully grasped or not retained information relating to placement, progress, arrangements, etc.

### Psychological well-being

*Assessment*
Peter presents as emotionally labile, depressed, with pain and fatigue. He is on high doses of antidepressant medication. The clinical questions are around adequate assessment of his mood and suicide risk, and evaluation of the therapeutic options in terms of treatment for his mood disorder.

Standardised mood questionnaires were considered and rejected as unhelpful in this case. Questionnaires with a significant language component and/or questions relating to pain or fatigue were not appropriate. Visual analogue scales were considered but it was decided that the level of explanation required was too great and that Peter would struggle to comprehend the instructions. Non-standardised assessment was complicated by the need to interpret Peter's gestures, which at times could be dramatic. For example, when asked about his future, or about his feelings, he would make an explicit gesture of cutting his throat. Staff and relatives found this gesture distressing and of concern. It is of particular relevance in Peter's case because it had been suggested that his injuries were secondary to a failed suicide attempt.

It was decided to use staff ratings of mood based on observable criteria such as level of interaction with staff and other clients, engagement with routine activities such as meals, social activities on the Unit, etc. Staff were asked to rate Peter's mood on a 1–10 scale at four points during the day. Over a period of weeks these observations showed a consistent pattern of low ratings for mood on waking, improvement at lunchtime and further improvement by teatime and evening. This pattern was consistent over many weeks although Peter's mood did vary over time, i.e. there were some days when his mood does not increase as much as on others but it did always show the same pattern of improvement once he was up and moving. Throughout this time his medication regime remained stable so there was no confounding effect of changes in antidepressant medication.

*Intervention*
Analysis of the records showed such a clear pattern of improved mood throughout the day that it was felt essential to use this information to change Peter's routine and avoid letting him spend long periods in bed. It was clear that this was detrimental to his mood. It was agreed to set up a behavioural

contract with Peter to encourage him to get up before 10 am. Implementing this was particularly difficult for the support staff as each morning Peter presented with low mood and distress, and it was hard for the staff to avoid being drawn into this and to remain focused on the need to encourage Peter to get up. However, with evidence from the recordings, especially when these were presented in a visual format, it was possible for them to reinforce the message to Peter each morning of the benefits of the programme.

The mood monitoring also showed that Peter's mood improved in relation to particular social activities and outings. Peter did not initiate any of these activities or show greater enthusiasm for them over others when he was offered them, but over time it has been possible to build up a clearer picture of which activities to encourage him in. There are particular activities that consistently raise his mood as measured by his level of engagement with the activity, a more animated facial expression and his willingness to engage with staff and others rather than retreat to his room. It has therefore been possible to programme in preferred activities and be firm in encouraging Peter to participate in spite of his tendency to refuse all activities when initially offered.

Consideration was given to the role Peter's gestures play in expressing his feelings. Attempts to explore these areas directly with him were distressing for him and he became more agitated as he perseverated on specific gestures, drawings or words on the page. The strategies that usually helped him to convey his meaning in day-to-day situations could not cope with these more abstract concepts. Over time and with a greater understanding of the diurnal variability in his mood, it was identified that his dramatic gestures occur in response to particular situations and reflect a high level of distress, but are not thought to be indicative of active suicidal ideation or intent. In reaching this conclusion Peter's general lack of initiation was a factor, as well as the contin- ued observations of his interactions with others and engagement in activities around the time he uses these gestures. The management approach taken to support Peter in his psychological well-being was to continue to provide positive experiences and to help Peter to engage with these wherever possible.

---

**Case Study 3.3  Aphasia and the use of counselling or psychological support**

*Brief history*
Martin is a 38-year-old man who sustained his brain injury in an assault 18 months ago. He was hit on the left side of his head with an iron bar and sustained a skull fracture and intracranial haemorrhage. Fragments of bone were embedded in brain tissue and it was necessary therefore to carry out a partial left frontal lobotomy. Following the attack, Martin is independently mobile but has no functional use of his right arm.

*Communication abilities*
Martin is aphasic with no meaningful verbal utterances. He cannot use writing but can match words to pictures although he rarely chooses to do so. He has a communication aid in the form of a personal digital assistant (PDA), which he does not use unless prompted. He can communicate his basic needs through gesture and facial expression. His comprehension of day-to-day activities and

conversations is good, as demonstrated by his ability to follow instructions and to carry out tasks. He is able to contribute to and join in group and social activities using his non-verbal skills.

*Psychological well-being*

Just prior to his injury, Martin and his wife had separated and the arrangements for access to their two young children are not yet finalised. This has clearly been causing distress and frustration for Martin, which he expressed by withdrawal from activities and by the use of non-verbal gestures. Whilst Martin is able to communicate successfully about his basic needs using his non-verbal skills, it is more difficult to assess and work with Martin at a more emotional level. On his PDA he has access to a range of emotional phrases and pictures, but he does not initiate using these even when he is clearly frustrated or upset.

It is therefore very difficult to know how to access Martin's emotional state or to support him in articulating his views about what he wants to happen. Like Peter in Case study 3.2, Martin can and does use dramatic and powerful gestures to express distress in broad terms, but lacks the communicative ability to work therapeutically to unpack these emotions. The work to help him understand the issues and then to support him working through how he feels and what decisions he wants to take is time consuming and sensitive, whether it is attempted using his PDA or on pen and paper. Apart from the practical difficulty of reducing complicated questions about child support arrangements or disposing of the family home to simple visual constructs, considerable care must be taken to provide open-ended questions and constructs to explore Martin's emotional state and not to direct or lead his responses. In more traditional psychotherapy it is often helpful to use metaphors and analogies to draw out different approaches to tasks or to explore previous ways of coping with difficult situations and look for parallels and differences with the current situation. Both of these approaches are of limited value with Martin. His communication impairment means that he cannot initiate sharing personal experiences with his therapist. His personal situation is such that the people who know him best, such as his wife or brother, and who could possibly have worked with him and a therapist in joint sessions, are not able to participate. With little or no access to his previous experiences, some examples can be sought from within the current environment but these are of little relevance to his family situation and can serve only to increase his annoyance both with his failure to communicate successfully and with the situation he finds himself in. The extent to which other cognitive deficits, including executive and memory difficulties, are also having an impact on his thinking and emotional responses is difficult to assess. Observation suggests that memory for day-to-day events and routines is reasonably good but that there is an element of rigidity in his behaviour that may also be affecting his thinking style. Ultimately it is a slow process and one that must be handled with sensitivity. Taking time to approach the issues on different occasions and looking for consistency over time is important in terms of the validity of any decisions Martin makes, but discussions about emotional adjustment may not be consistent over time, and it is important but not easy to separate practical decision making from psychological adjustment.

## Summary

People with communication impairment as part of an acquired brain injury have a particularly difficult set of challenges to face in terms of their psychological well-being. Their access to therapy may be reduced and this can have a direct effect on their psychological well-being through a reduced ability to be supported to work through emotional issues, and an indirect impact as their opportunities for normal positive engagement with the world and positive feedback through everyday activities are also reduced. Recognising these challenges and providing staff support and time to seek to address them is the challenge facing brain injury services.

## References

Aben I, Verhey F, Honig A, Lodder J, Lousberg R, Maes M. Research into the specificity of depression after stroke: A review on an unresolved issue. Progr Neuro-psychoph 2001;25:671–689.

Bennett HE, Thomas SA, Austen R, Morris AMS, Lincoln NB. Validation of screening measures for assessing mood in stroke patients. Brit J Clin Psychol 2006;45:367–376.

Bennett TL. Individual psychotherapy and minor head injury. Cogn Rehabil 1989;Sep/Oct: 20–25.

Bond M. The psychiatry of closed head injury. In: Brooks N (ed.) Closed Head Injury. Psychological, Social and Family Consequences. London: Oxford University Press, 1984; pp. 148–178.

Brooks DN, McKinley WW. Personality and behavioural change after severe blunt head injury—a relative's view. J Neurol Neurosur Ps 1983;46:336–344.

Brumfitt SM, Sheeran P. The development and validation of the Visual Analogue Self-Esteem Scale (VASES). Brit J Clin Psychol 1999;38:387–400.

Douglas JM, Spellacy FJ. Indicators of long term family functioning following severe traumatic brain injury in adults. Brain Injury 1996;10:819–839.

Douglas JM, O'Flaherty C, Snow P. Measuring perception of communicative ability: The development and evaluation of the La Trobe Communication Questionnaire. Aphasiology 2000;14:251–268.

Ellis DW. Foundation of Neuropsychology Series: Neuropsychotherapy. Neuropsychological Treatment after Brain Injury. Boston: Kluwer, 1989; pp. 241–269.

Evans JJ, Levine B. Mood disorders: Issues of prevalence, misdiagnosis, assessment, and treatment. Neuropsychol Rehabil 2002;12:167–170.

Fleminger S, Oliver DL, Williams WH, Evans J. The neuropsychiatry of depression after brain injury. Neuropsychol Rehabil 2003;13:65–87.

Gainotti G. Emotional and psychosocial problems after brain injury. Neuropsychol Rehabil 1993;3:259–277.

Gervasio AH, Kreutzer JS. Kinship and family members' psychological distress after traumatic brain injury: A large sample study. J Head Trauma Rehab 1997;12:14–26.

Gillen R, Tennen H, Affleck G, Steinpreis R. Distress, depressive symptoms and depressive disorder among caregivers of patients with brain injury. J Head Trauma Rehab 1998;13:31–43.

Gosling J, Oddy M. Rearranged marriages: marital relationships after head injury. Brain Injury 1999;13:785–796.

Jennett B, MacMillan R. Epidemiology of head injury. BMJ 1981;282:101–104.

Kreutzer JS, Gervasio AH, Camplair PS. Primary caregivers' psychological status and family functioning after traumatic brain injury. Brain Injury 1994;8:197–210.

Lewis L. A framework for developing a psychotherapy treatment plan with brain-injured patients. J Head Trauma Rehab 1991;6:22–29.

Lezak MD. Living with the characterologically altered brain injured patient. J Clin Psychiat 1978;39:592–598.

Livingston MG, Brooks DN. The burden on families of the brain injured: A review. J Head Trauma Rehab 1988;3:6–15.

Malec J. Training the brain-injured client in behavioural self-management skills. In: Edelstein BA, Couture ET (eds) Behaviour Assessment and Rehabilitation of Traumatically Brain Damaged Adults. New York: Plenum Press, 1994; pp. 121–150.

McMillan TM. Neuropsychological assessment after extremely severe head injury in a case of life or death. Brain Injury 1996;11:483–490.

McMillan TM, Herbert CM. Neuropsychological assessment of a possible 'euthanasia' case: a 5 year follow up. Brain Injury 2000;14:197–203.

McMillan TM, Herbert CM. Further recovery in a potential treatment withdrawal case 10 years after brain injury. Brain Injury 2004;18:935–940.

Moore AD, Stambrook M, Peters LC, Lubusko A. Family coping and marital adjustment after traumatic brain injury. J Head Trauma Rehab 1991;6:83–89.

Nadell J. Towards an existential psychotherapy with the traumatically injured brain injured patient. Cogn Rehabil 1991;13:8–13.

Neurological Alliance. Neuronumbers—a Brief Review of the Numbers of People in the UK with a Neurological Condition. London: Neurological Alliance, 2003.

Oddy M. He's no longer the same person: How families adjust to personality change after head injury. In: Chamberlain MA, Neumann V, Tennant A (eds) Traumatic Brain Injury Rehabilitation. London: Chapman and Hall, 1995; pp. 167–180.

Oddy M, Herbert CM. Intervention with families following brain injury: Evidence-based practice. Neuropsychol Rehabil 2003;13:259–273.

Oddy M, Humphrey M, Uttley D. Stresses upon the relatives of head-injured patients. Brit J Psychiat 1978;133:507–513.

Oddy M, Coughlan T, Tyerman A, Jenkins D et al. Social adjustment after closed head injury: a further follow-up seven years after injury. J Neurol Neurosur Ps 1985;48:564–568.

Perlesz A, Furlong M, McLachlan D. Family-centred rehabilitation: Family Therapy for the head injured and their relatives. In: Harris R, Burns R, Rees R (eds) Recovery from Brain Injury: Expectations, Needs and Processes. Adelaide: Institute for the Study of Learning Difficulties, 1989; pp. 180–191.

Perlesz A, Kinsella G, Crowe S. Impact of traumatic brain injury on the family: A critical review. Rehabil Psychol 1999;44:6–35.

Prigatano GP. Disordered mind, wounded soul: The emerging role of psychotherapy in rehabilitation after brain injury. J Head Trauma Rehab 1991;6:1–10.

Sparadeo FD, Strauss D, Barth JT. The incidence, impact, and treatment of substance abuse in head trauma rehabilitation. J Head Trauma Rehab 1990;5:1–8.

Stern RA, Arruda JE, Hooper CR, Wolfner GD, Morey CE. Visual analogue mood scales to measure internal mood state in neurologically impaired patients: description and initial validity evidence. Aphasiology 1997;11: 59–71.

Sutcliffe LM, Lincoln NB. The assessment of depression in aphasic stroke patients: development of the Stroke Aphasic Depression Questionnaire. Clin Rehabil 1998;12:506–513.

Tate RL. Beyond one-bun two-shoe: Recent advances in the psychological rehabilitation of memory disorders after acquired brain injury. Brain Injury 1997;11:907–918.

Taylor LA, Kreutzer JS, Demm SR, Meade MA. Traumatic brain injury and substance abuse: A review and analysis of the literature. Neuropsychol Rehabil 2003;13:165–188.

Teasdale TW, Engberg AW. Suicide after traumatic brain injury: A population study. J Neurol Neurosur Ps 2001;71:436–440.

Tennant A. Admission to hospital following head injury in England: Incidence and socio-economic associations. BMC Public Health 2005;21:(5).

Thomsen IV. Late outcome of very severe blunt head trauma: a 10–15 year second follow-up. J Neurol Neurosur Ps 1984;47:260–268.

Thornhill S, Teasdale GM, Murray GD, McEwen J, Roy CW, Penny KI. Disability in young people and adults one year after head injury: prospective cohort study. BMJ 2000;320: 1631–1635.

Turner-Stokes L, Kalmus M, Hirani D, Clegg F. The depression intensity scale circles (DISCs): a first evaluation of a simple assessment tool for depression in the context of brain injury. J Neurol Neurosur Ps 2005;76:1273–1278.

Wallace CA, Bogner J, Corrigan JD, Clinchot D, Mysiw WJ, Fugate LP. Primary caregivers of persons with brain injury: Life change 1 year after injury. Brain Injury 1998;12:483–493.

Watkins C, Leathley M, Daniels L, Dickinson H, Lightbody CE, van den Broek M, Jack CIA. The Signs of Depression Scale in stroke: how useful are nurses' observations? Clin Rehabil 2001;15:447–457.

Williams WH, Williams JMG, Ghadiali EJ. Autobiographical memory in traumatic brain injury: Neuropsychological and mood predictors of recall. Neuropsychol Rehabil 1998;8: 43–60.

Youngson H, Alderman N. Fear of incontinence and its effects on a community based rehabilitation after severe brain injury: Successful remediation of escape behaviour using behaviour modification. Brain Injury 1992;10:229–238.

# 4 The Role of Self-Esteem: Issues in Acquired Communication Impairments

### Shelagh Brumfitt

## Introduction

Self-esteem is a term that is frequently used in everyday conversation but also used within a formal framework of psychological terminology. There has been a limited interest in this aspect of the individual experience in the clinical conditions that are related to acquired communication impairments, such as stroke and head injury. This is surprising, given the focus in our society on the importance of self-worth.

In Western societies self-esteem is generally viewed as an important component in how an individual copes in society. Low self-esteem is frequently perceived as the cause of individual social impairments, examples including addictive behaviours where individuals might drink to overcome feelings of low self-worth. Blascovich and Tomaka (1991) state: 'self esteem is the extent to which one prizes, values, approves or likes oneself' (p. 115). Within the social psychological literature, self-esteem is usually described as the overall evaluation of one's worth. It involves the value an individual places on self. It is generally seen as a core feature of the self concept. Santrock (2001) defines self-esteem as 'the global evaluative dimension of the self' (p. 302): that is, the individual will have feelings about the self that are positive or negative (e.g. I'm responsible, not responsible; I'm clever, not clever), and that will influence self-worth. The evaluations of all of the personal attributes that individuals may use about themselves create overall self-esteem. In general, it is considered that self-esteem and knowledge of self builds up over time and becomes relatively stable, although self-esteem will be vulnerable to various factors. Trait self-esteem is considered to be an enduring characteristic of the person's personality, but self-esteem can also show short-term variations that are affected by immediate experiences, and this is often referred to as state self-esteem.

Harter (1993) argues that the origin of self-esteem has two sources. The first is that of the direct experience of competence or efficacy, where individuals can recognise valuable qualities or effectiveness in themselves.

The second source is from social feedback, where the individual uses the perceived evaluations of others to influence levels of self-esteem. This may begin in the early years in the close family context. Self-esteem may also be influenced by social comparison (Festinger, 1954). Social comparisons refer to the process of comparing one's own self (e.g. one aspect of self, such as professional ability) with those of other people. Although individuals do not consciously compare themselves with everyone they meet, there are times when they may compare themselves with someone they know well who is working in the same context, for example. Self-esteem may be influenced by the views of a close friend or if there is a dimension of comparison that is perceived as very important. Perhaps a work colleague achieves a task to a much higher standard than another person and is rewarded for that. There is the potential for changes to self-esteem in these colleagues, and these self-views may be maintained over time if the two colleagues continue to work together. Alternatively, self-esteem is unlikely to be affected by the accomplishments of people individuals do not know well, although some individuals will make comparisons between themselves and famous people, and a proportion will find these comparisons influence their level of self-esteem. Cant (1997) notes that during his recovery from a stroke, he became aware that he was using other patients as reference points to compare his own recovery with theirs. He reported that he became concerned if he saw someone walking or using their damaged hand before he could and noted that he believed it affected his self-esteem.

Self-esteem may be influenced by longstanding cognitions about the self. For example, believing one's self to be a hopeless athlete may be part of one's self-image but not bear any relation to self-worth (because being an athlete does not rate as important for that individual). However, if being good at athletics was an important aspect of an individual's life, this *would* link into feelings of self-worth or self-esteem.

Self-esteem is usually considered as a global construct rather than specific, although individuals will have evaluations about a particular dimension, such as physical self-worth or academic self-worth. A key assumption is that variations in self-esteem can influence outcomes, such as whether someone becomes an alcoholic or makes repeated suicide attempts. Self-esteem could therefore be potentially used as a marker or a predictor of outcome. So, for professionals in mental health contexts, concerns will focus on whether levels of self-esteem make these sort of outcomes more or less likely. Self-esteem has certainly been implicated in depression, suicide, delinquency and anorexia (Santrock, 2001). Also, self-esteem may be considered as an outcome itself, what different experiences may potentially contribute to self-esteem, such as loss of employment and, possibly, stroke and aphasia.

There is a psychological view also, that most people will desire to achieve maximum feelings of self-worth, although there is some recent evidence that people with low self-esteem may be resistant to change (Josephs, Bosson and Jacobs, 2003). Tesser (1995), in a review of self-esteem research, notes that low self-esteem does not appear to be the perception that the self is worthless, rather it is the absence of reasons for believing that the self has value. That is, low self-esteem has been associated with poorly developed notions of the self, so that self-understanding may be more limited than in the person with high self-esteem. Thus, trying to increase self-esteem in the low self-esteem individual may also prove more difficult because the confused and poorly defined self-views are more difficult to elaborate.

This may have implications for how we consider the language-impaired speaker. Would the loss of language mean that self descriptions become less well defined and therefore have an influence on self-worth?

## Society's influence on self-esteem

Marmot (2003) argues that in a society that is full of inequality, there will be some inequalities that are the result of variations in self-esteem. That is, the individual's self-perception may contribute to the way a society functions, because an individual with low self-esteem may behave differently to an individual with higher self-esteem. According to Marmot, these inequalities in self-esteem have a relationship to health status, hence self-esteem merits further attention in the healthcare context. Krause and Alexander (1990) investigated the relationship of psychological distress in later life with self-esteem and noted that appropriate levels of self-esteem enable the individual to use an 'active problem solving approach to resolving stressful circumstances' (p. 420). The implication is that individuals with appropriate levels of self-esteem are more likely to be able to be self-reliant within their own social context and cope better as they age.

In relation to demographic factors in self-esteem, Emler (2001) reported that there was little evidence for a relationship between membership of an ethnic group and self-esteem. Given that membership of certain ethnic groups may imply discrimination, the research in this area shows surprisingly little evidence for it impacting upon levels of self-esteem (Gray-Little and Hafdahl, 2000). Social class position is related to adult self-esteem but, according to Emler's review, in only a modest way. Furthermore, gender has not been found to show a strong relationship with self-esteem, although like these other factors, it would be easy to assume that they were strongly related. The key aspect of our human experience in relation to our level of self-esteem appears to be the influence of our parents. Emler (2001) quotes research by Katz (2000), which shows that paternal support and interest is critical in sustaining the self-esteem of sons who are moving through adolescence.

## Depression and self-esteem

There is clearly some association between depression and self-esteem. Typically, an individual who scores highly on self-esteem will score low on depression and vice versa. Arguments have been made for the two being part of the same overall state. Tennen and Affleck (1993) argue that depression, as a clinical state that needs medical attention and medication, is qualitatively different to self-esteem. People do not get admitted to hospital for low self-esteem, for example. Emler (2001) concludes that there is an overlap, with the two states sharing some attributes while maintaining others that are distinct. Methods for examining psychological well-being generally include measures of both, confirming therefore that they are two distinct states that can be measured separately. Debate in the professional and academic literature exists about whether changes in self-esteem cause depression or whether low self-esteem is a result of depression. As yet there is no definitive answer to this, and it may be the case that they influence each other.

Vickery, Sepehri and Evans (2008) report a large study comparing ratings of self-esteem and depressive mood in a sample of 80 stroke survivors referred for neuropsychological evaluation, with a matched control group. The stroke group were admitted to rehabilitation approximately 14 days after admission to hospital following stroke, and the data was therefore collected (3–25 days following entry to the rehabilitation programme) at a relatively early stage in their recovery period. Participants were asked to complete the Visual Analogue Self-esteem Scale (VASES; Brumfitt and Sheeran, 1999a), the Rosenberg Self-esteem Scale (Rosenberg, 1965) and the Geriatric Depression Scale (Yesavage *et al.*, 1983). The results showed that when the individual items on the VASES were compared between the two groups, the stroke survivors rated themselves as being less cheerful and intelligent, and more mixed up, trapped and frustrated than the control group. This group of stroke survivors also indicated significantly greater levels of depression than the control group when measured on the Geriatric Depression Scale. Overall, their findings indicate that lowered self-esteem is associated with effects of stroke, and direct work on raising self-esteem post-stroke is a potential intervention strategy.

## Can self-esteem be changed?

One of the key beliefs about self-esteem is that low self-esteem is bad and high self-esteem is good. As Emler (2001) reasons, this is more complicated than first appears. If self-esteem is low, is there a moral imperative to change this? What are the characteristics of an individual with low self-esteem? Are the people with low self-esteem always members of groups who have significant impairments in society or is it possible to function relatively well in society but still have low self-esteem?

Some of the work looking at the significance of low or high self-esteem has come from marketing and advertising. One presupposition is that a person with low self-esteem is more likely to be easily influenced than someone with high self-esteem. That is, if an individual sees himself as unattractive he may be more likely to spend money on goods that persuade him that this will make a difference to his attractiveness. Rhodes and Wood (1992) demonstrated that extremes of self-esteem levels were less easy to change, as evidenced in their meta-analysis of research on self-esteem and tendency to conform and tendency to be influenced. That is, it was the people with moderate self-esteem scores who showed most inclination to conform or be influenced. It was suggested that people with low self-esteem have difficulty receiving whatever is given to them to help them change; and people with high self-esteem are also unlikely to conform because they do not see the need to take notice. In addition, if we accept Tesser's (1995) view of this, about trying to increase self-esteem in the low self-esteem individual, may also prove more difficult because they have more confused and poorly defined self-views that are known to be more difficult to elaborate, even with specific help.

There are differences in the way that self-esteem functions as an outcome in therapeutic interventions. Essentially, there are two models. Firstly, that of broad-based therapy where self-esteem is one outcome alongside others such as levels of depression and anxiety. An example of this might be direct speech and language therapy for speech intelligibility for people with dysarthria. Evaluations would include a pre- and post-therapy measure of self-esteem, as well as a pre- and post-therapy measure of intelligibility and a pre- and post-therapy measure of communicative effectiveness. Here the speech and language therapist is looking for outcome across a set of different dimensions. Alternatively, enhancing self-esteem may be the main objective of the therapy, and changes to the level of self-esteem may be the only outcome required. Of the small amount of work on self-esteem in aphasia, none has been directed at raising self-esteem specifically, thus the results on change to self-esteem that exist in the literature are based on research that has other outcomes also. However, reports on interventions in other areas such as learning disability are relevant here and comparisons can be made. Whelan, Haywood and Galloway (2007) described a group of people with learning disability who worked specifically on low self-esteem by using cognitive behaviour therapy. Here the aim of the group was to improve self-esteem by working on cognitions associated with low self-esteem, such as perceptions of capacity to get needs met, perceived and real deficiencies in social networks, and the influence social comparison factors. In order to demonstrate outcome, a modified version of the Rosenberg Self-esteem Scale (1965) was used (Figure 4.1), which simplified the language and provided a colour cue method for responses. Out of the five members of the group two members showed improved self-esteem scores over the course of 10 weekly sessions. Although this is a different population and there are limited changes demonstrated, the approach has the potential for use in the acquired populations.

|  | Strongly agree | Agree | Disagree | Strongly disagree |
|---|---|---|---|---|
| I feel that I'm a person of worth, at least on an equal plane with others |  |  |  |  |
| I feel that i have a number of good qualities |  |  |  |  |
| All in all, I'm inclined to feel that I'm a failure** |  |  |  |  |
| I am able to do things as well as most other people |  |  |  |  |
| I feel I do not have much to be proud of ** |  |  |  |  |
| I take a positive attitude toward myself |  |  |  |  |
| On the whole, I am satisfied with myself |  |  |  |  |
| I wish I could have more respect for myself ** |  |  |  |  |
| I certainly feel useless at times ** |  |  |  |  |
| At times I think I am no good at all ** |  |  |  |  |

Scoring: remove asterisks when administering.
For items 1,2,4,6,7: strongly agree = 3, agree = 2, disagree = 1 and strongly disagree = 0.
For items 3,5,8,9,10 (which are reversed in valence and noted with asterisks**) reverse the scoring.

**Figure 4.1** The Rosenberg Self Esteem Scale (Rosenberg, 1965). Reproduced with permission of The Morris Rosenberg Foundation.

## Self-esteem in people with disability

The role of self-esteem in relation to disability is not fully understood, but there is a developing and expanding literature. Evidence from different clinical populations reveals what the main issues are and directs clinical approaches towards areas where effectiveness has been shown. It is probably true to say that on clinical intuition alone a health professional would expect that having a disability would create low self-esteem in the individual. Cant (1997), in a personal account of his stroke, notes that the speech and language therapy he received was more stressful than any of the other therapies, and puts forward a hypothesis that self-esteem is more damaged by loss of speaking ability then any other impact of stroke. However, the literature does not show a clear-cut association.

Although no difference was found between the self-esteem scores of 25 elementary school children who stuttered and the normative data,

Yovetich, Leschied and Flicht (2000) discuss the reasons why this should be. One of their suggestions is that the measures used are not suitable for people who stutter because they do not capture the construct of self as a speaker. Finding and using appropriate measures for the communicatively impaired speaker is of critical importance if accurate understanding is to be gained.

Much of the work that is done on self-esteem has been based upon the experience of young people. Manuel *et al.* (2003) reported a study that examined predictors of self-esteem in 50 older children and young people with cerebral palsy. Based on the results from the Rosenberg Self-esteem Scale (1965) these participants had mean self-esteem scores comparable with samples of healthy adults and young adults with chronic illness. The authors discuss this finding and conclude that physical disability is not necessarily associated with low self-esteem in young people. Westbrook, Bauman and Shinnar (1992) examined social stigma in young people with chronic conditions. Using 64 young people with epilepsy, they looked at the relationships between perceptions of stigma, how individuals disclosed their medical conditions and levels of self esteem. The results revealed that seizure type and participant's belief that the epilepsy was a stigmatising condition predicted poor self-esteem.

>McAndrew (1999) looked at whether high levels of emotional and behavioural impairments in language-disordered children were associated with low self-esteem in a small sample of 14 children. No association was found but the author noted that some of the children had difficulty understanding the meaning of the questions in the scales used: the Piers–Harris Children's Self-Concept Scale and the Coopersmith Inventory. This may have influenced the results. Subsequently, Jerome, Fujiki, Brinton and James (2002) explored the self-esteem of children with specific language impairment (SLI) in comparison to those with typical development. Because the characteristics of communication impairment mean that there will be educational and social implications for a child who has SLI, it was hypothesised that these children would be vulnerable to low self-esteem. Two groups of children were examined; 46 between the ages of 6 and 9, and 34 between the ages of 10 and 13. In the younger group, there were no statistically significant differences were demonstrated between children with SLI and typically developing children in relation to perceived competence and acceptance. However, in the older group, children with SLI perceived themselves more negatively in scholastic competence, social acceptance and behavioural conduct than did those children who were in the group of typically developing children. The authors suggest that the risk for low self-esteem increases as the child enters middle to late childhood and becomes more aware of differences between self and others.

In order to understand more about the subjective experiences of people with schizophrenia, Sörgaard *et al.* (2002) examined self-esteem in random samples of people with schizophrenia receiving outpatient services in 10 psychiatric centres in five Nordic countries (Norway, Finland, Sweden, Denmark, Iceland). The variations in self-esteem were found to be most associated with differences in anxiety and depression and reported satisfaction with family relationships. Having at least one friend was the strongest social network predictor. The authors note that clinical management of anxiety and depression may be of importance in enhancing self-esteem, and that the quality of the health service system for dealing with this problem may be influential. There is also some evidence to show that service intensity and length of time of services were associated with improvements of self-esteem in a group of persons with schizophrenia.

Chang and Mackenzie (1998) examined state self-esteem after stroke in 152 patients following admission and up to 3 months after admission. Although a test of depression was not used, the Heatherton and Polivy State Self-esteem Scale (Heatherton and Polivy, 1991) and the Rosenberg Self-esteem (RSE) Scale (1965) were used. According to the results, state self-esteem was significantly correlated with functional independence. The authors suggest that levels of self-esteem can influence outcome, and note that more study is needed to look at the use of psychosocial interventions in reducing the threat to self from stroke and the effect on functional outcome.

## The measurement of self-esteem

Self-esteem has traditionally been measured by using self-report scales, although some reference is made by Emler (2001) of approaches that have been tried using observational methods of behaviour, where another person rates an individual's self-esteem. Because of unreliability of observer ratings, self-report is most commonly used as it can then access the individual's internal feelings. Yet, it has to be acknowledged that self-report, as a process, is rarely unpicked to examine what components make up the individual's capacity to do this. In a textbook of long standing, Burns (1979) described the following factors as influencing whether an individual was able to self-report.

- the clarity of the individual's awareness;
- the availability of adequate symbols for expression;
- the willingness of the individual to co-operate;
- social expectancy;
- the individual's feeling of inadequacy;
- his feelings of freedom from threat (p. 75).

Clearly the 'availability of adequate symbols for expression' recognises the role of speech and language in this process.

For the person with aphasia, this creates some challenges. Looking firstly to the existing scales developed for the population where speech and language is assumed to be intact, a typical example of a measure of self-esteem is Rosenberg's scale (1965) (see Figure 4.1), which is widely used and highly valued because of its simplicity. The scale consists of 10 statements, five of which are phrased in the positive direction (e.g. 'I feel that I'm a person of worth, at least on an equal plane with others') and five that are negatively phrased (e.g. 'All in all I am inclined to feel I'm a failure'). The statements are rated on a four-point scale ranging from 'strongly agree' to 'strongly disagree'. The validity of the RSE is well established and is frequently used in research. However, it can be seen from the examples given that the statements require linguistic comprehension in order for the respondent to self-report using this scale. Of all the methods to use, self-report is the one that is likely to cause the most difficulty for a person with aphasia because of the reliance on language. The literature acknowledges this. Starkstein and Robinson (1988) described the emotional reactions to aphasia but also noted the difficulties in assessing these: 'The single greatest obstacle is the fundamental paradox of studying a problem (i.e. emotional disorder) when the basic method for assessing the problem (i.e. language) is disturbed' (p. 1).

Later, Gainotti (1997) also examined the emotional, psychological and psychosocial impairments of aphasic patients and noted the limited attention given to these in research: 'This paradoxical state of affairs is due both to the extreme complexity of this field of investigation and to the poverty of research tools enabling investigators to explore it effectively' (p. 635).

What aspects are important in understanding the written word in traditional self-report scales? Items or statements that the individual has to understand before being able to respond appropriately need a critical evaluation. One example from a depression scale uses symbolic language (e.g. 'I feel downhearted and blue'; Zung, Richards, Gables and Short, 1965). Symbolic language is very difficult for an aphasic speaker or speaker with head injury, and there is the risk that the speaker would interpret this statement in a concrete literal manner. General readability therefore needs to be taken into account when developing self-report scales, although many of those previously published have not done so. In a systematic review of the diagnosis of depression in people with aphasia, Townend, Brady and McLoughlan (2007) noted that 48% of 60 studies indicated that they had adapted the method for diagnosis to take account of the language impairments in the participants. The types of adaptive methods used included using informants, clinical observation, modifying questions or responses required, or changing the timing of the interviews to take account of recovery periods or using visual analogue scales.

General understanding about accessibility to diagnostic scales and any sort of written material uses the concept of readability to determine how well a person can access material. Readability reflects the simplicity of the written text. It is partly determined by sentence length, and clearly, for aphasic and head-injured speakers, the length should be short.

Rose *et al.* (2003) shortened sentences to an average of 6.6 to 9.1 words for aphasic speakers. Passive sentences are also to be avoided as meaning cannot be determined through word order. High-frequency words are also recommended for use, as are high-imageability words.

Starkstein and Robinson (1988) noted that the methods by which understanding of self-esteem emerges in aphasic people, for example, has therefore rested upon the development of scales that are not completely language dependent. There has been little to use in the past, but more recently, as a response to this problem, the Visual Analogue Self-esteem Scale (VASES; Brumfitt and Sheeran, 1999b) was developed and has provided a method for assessing self-esteem in aphasic people. The scale consists of 10 paired items, which have written and picture representations, and therefore permit the respondent to have an enhanced understanding of the meaning of the item. The response scale also uses visual images to support understanding. The VASES has good demonstrated reliability and validity (Brumfitt and Sheeran, 1999b). Thus a reliable assessment of self-esteem can now be obtained from a large proportion of aphasic speakers and used in both the research and rehabilitative contexts. The scores used can show individual change over time, with a highest score of 50 and a lowest score of 10. There are no cut-off scores to provide a diagnosis, but clearly a low score of self-esteem is likely to indicate the risk of depression.

Vickery (2006) investigated the use of the VASES in 156 acute-phase stroke survivors in order to determine whether the VASES was useful in this type of population. Factors affecting the suitability of the VASES were examined by looking at variables such as visual acuity, the nature of the aphasia and visuo-perceptual deficits. The impact of other characteristics was also examined, such as demographic variables, prior stroke, stroke laterality and cognitive functioning. Levels of distress were also measured. From the results, Vickery was able to show that the VASES is not affected by cognitive functioning, lower visual acuity or visuo-perceptual involvement. No significant correlations between the demographic characteristics of age, race, gender and education were found. Patients with the most severe language impairments were found to be less able to respond appropriately to the picture stimuli of the VASES. Vickery reports that patients appeared to select the positive stimuli if they were in the most severe language-impaired category, which suggests that the purpose of the task may have been misunderstood. Vickery cautions against the use of the VASES for severely impaired aphasic speakers. However, this study also demonstrated the usefulness of the VASES for identifying patients with high risk for emotional dysfunction. The correlations between self-esteem ratings on the VASES and measures of depression and anxiety and overall emotional distress were significant. Vickery also recommends the use of the VASES for the general stroke population.

In a study looking at the validity of screening measures for assessing mood in stroke patients (Bennett *et al.*, 2006), 50 healthy older adults and

100 stroke patients in hospital completed a range of tests of well-being in order to establish which were suitable to use as screening tests of mood after stroke. The authors concluded that the VASES was a useful measure for monitoring mood over time and evaluating the outcome of interventions, but less useful for screening purposes.

## Methods for evaluating self-esteem in people with acquired communication impairments

It is particularly the acquired language-impaired group for whom there is a need to overcome barriers to comprehension of language in measurement scales. Most of the focus has been on aphasia, where there is evidence of literature that considers appropriate methodologies. People with dementia form another population for whom cognitive and language impairments create significant barriers to comprehension. The essential challenge facing the health professional is to find a way of obtaining an understanding about an individual's self-view in these conditions.

One possible solution is to try to create an alternative route to understanding that avoids the focus on language. The use of picture material is the most obvious alternative method. However, in order to make use of picture material, the meaning of the picture has to be very clear, otherwise the picture will create confusion rather than enhance understanding. The literature on self-evaluation of pain provides some good guidance (pain assessment tools: http://www.npci.org.uk/therapeutics/pain/otherback/resources/pda_pain_overview.pdf; accessed 28 May 2009).

In terms of making written materials aphasia friendly, pictures are often recommended (Pound, Parr and Woolf, 2000). However, the use of pictures needs further elaboration. There is a risk that adults may be unhappy about pictures, believing this may trivialise important issues (Rees, Ford and Sheard, 2003). Houts, Doak, Doak and Loscalzo (2006) provide an extensive review of the role of pictures in improving health communication. Research evidence suggests that pictures do aid comprehension. However, pictures can also interfere with comprehension. If the picture fails to help the reader understand the information or concept involved, it may instead create a further confusion. Some research has shown that amongst poor readers very detailed pictures can distract attention away from printed words because the reader starts to focus on irrelevant aspects (Houts, Doak, Doak and Loscalzo, 2006). Simple drawings appear to be the most effective in furthering understanding of a concept. Hoffman and Worrall (2004) recommend that for drawing to be useful (in health education contexts) it should only communicate one single idea. In practice this may not be so easy to achieve and pictures may vary in the complexity of what they portray. A picture of an animal conveys one basic concept. However, attempting to portray a complex abstract concept such as 'hope' or 'satisfaction' is much more difficult to achieve. In order to use the pictures in the VASES, for example, face and construct validity of the pictures had to be demonstrated (Brumfitt and Sheeran, 1999b). Originally there were 24 pairs of pictures, which had been drawn to represent the different aspects of the aphasic experience that had emerged from the literature and some early work (Brumfitt, 1985). Non-aphasic speakers were invited to examine the pictures and suggest their meanings. Not all of these were comprehensible to the participants who were involved in the face validity testing, and finding accessible picture material was challenging. For example, attempting to find a visual portrayal of 'optimistic' was difficult. This is a complex construct that is relevant and meaningful to people in rehabilitation, but there is no immediate visual image that comes to mind when thinking about feelings of optimism. Eventually, the decision to use the image of a cloud to represent 'not optimistic' and a rainbow to represent 'optimistic' was found to be recognisable (Figure 4.2).

Examples of pictures that had to be discarded in the development of the VASES are presented in Figures 4.3 and 4.4 to show the difficulties involved in designing suitable pictures. For Figure 4.3 the intention to portray 'competent' and 'not competent' was obscured by the literal interpretation of the pictures: that is, participants were drawn to seeing this as demonstrating something to do with the skill of erecting a tent. Similarly, in Figure 4.4 the intention to portray 'moody' and 'not moody' was extremely difficult to achieve. This picture did not put the concept across well and was clearly too complex in the face validity testing.

Other factors in relation to the use of pictures include potential difficulties for the neurologically impaired population, who may experience difficulties in visual processing. Furthermore, cultural relevance is another factor that may influence understanding and this needs to be taken into account when considering self-esteem ratings.

In addition to the use of pictures to represent the verbal items in a test, the response section of a test needs to take into account the linguistic ability

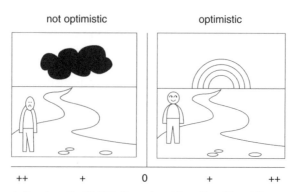

**Figure 4.2** Sample item from the VASES. Reproduced from Brumfitt and Sheeran (1999a), by kind permission of Speeechmark Publishing Limited.

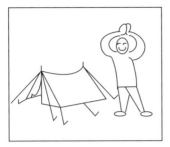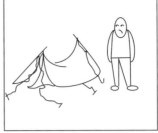

**Figure 4.3** Discarded pair of pictures used in original development work for VASES. The pictures were intended to show the concepts of 'competent' and 'not competent'.

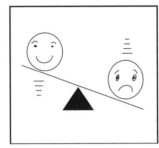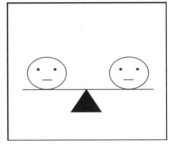

**Figure 4.4** Discarded pair of pictures used in original development work for VASES. The pictures were intended to show the concepts of 'moody' and 'not moody'.

of the respondent. A Likert scale usually includes a range of choices for the respondent to use; such as strongly agree, agree, undecided, disagree and strongly disagree (Bowling, 1997). Sometimes scales use wider ranges, such as a set of seven choices. The difficulty for the communicatively impaired speaker is that this requires a further task of linguistic analysis. The respondent needs to look at the test items (which may or may not be enhanced by the use of pictures), decide the meaning of the item and then decide which rating best reflects the self-view. Then the respondent has to indicate the rating, either by marking this or by having another person help. If the ratings include complex choices, then the self-view may be inaccurate because the respondent has been unable to complete the task because of the communication difficulty. Even a simple rating choice, such as true or false, may be demanding for someone with a language problem. Semantic confusions may arise and the result may not be representative of the 'real' self-view.

In developing the VASES it was important to find a rating scale that would help the respondent. Based on advice from professionals working with populations with learning difficulties, it was decided to use symbols for the rating procedure, as seen in Figure 4.5. Thus, only + and 0 were used, but in different combinations.

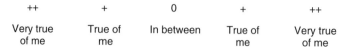

| ++ | + | 0 | + | ++ |
|---|---|---|---|---|
| Very true of me | True of me | In between | True of me | Very true of me |

**Figure 4.5** Symbols used for the rating procedure in VASES. Reproduced by permission of Speechmark Publishing Ltd.

This also removed the bias of producing a negative side to the pairs of pictures. For example, the respondent was only required to indicate whether they agreed with the description represented in the picture above. There was no need to indicate strong agreement or disagreement.

In the final version of the VASES the symbols are presented with the verbal labels, and they are placed immediately below each pair of pictures. The administering clinician is permitted to tell the client the meaning of each picture (i.e. it is not a task of language comprehension) and allow the individual time to look at the picture. Thus, helping the individual to understand the picture is acceptable. Obviously, what the clinician cannot do is direct the response to each pair of pictures.

The pairs of pictures are deliberately placed so that there is no regular configuration of negative pictures down one side of the page. The configuration is random. Thus no client can 'learn' to respond to a certain side on the sheet.

As more tests of self-esteem are developed there will be improvements to the existing formats, based on accumulated understanding from the evidence base. However, this is a particularly difficult area to work in because of the complexity of the conditions.

In order to find the best possible methods, it will be important to interact with other specialities that need to develop materials that are accessible to people with communication and cognitive disabilities.

## Self-esteem in aphasia

There is a recognition supported by evidence that the role of the 'self' in recovery from aphasia has significance (Brumfitt, 1993; Code, Helmsley and Herrman, 1999) and that association between self-image and communicative handicap should not be overlooked. Letourneau (1993) noted that aphasia causes damage to self-esteem and that 'sources of self confidence are temporarily blocked and some may never be reinstated' (p. 73). Regaining self-esteem after loss of communication may not be possible by the individual without professional help. Muller (1999) argued for merging psychosocial adjustment into treatment plans for people with aphasia. He stated: 'it is imperative therefore, that in evaluating the effectiveness of rehabilitation programmes in aphasia, consideration be given to self-esteem and that appropriate measures be incorporated into the programme' (p. 90). This had become an area of emerging interest.

In a survey of 173 speech and language therapists in the UK (Brumfitt, 2006), participants reported a wide range of materials for evaluating psychosocial status with aphasic speakers. Out of this set of participants, only 39% reported using published scales to examine psychosocial dimensions, and of this 39% only 15% reported using a measure of self-esteem. Clearly, these results only reflect the reported practice of a proportion of participants. However, the results do show that for a variety of possible reasons, self-esteem measures are not widely used and may confirm the commentaries by Gainotti (1997) and Starkstein and Robinson (1988) about the limited materials available.

However, the ways in which self-esteem is important to the individual experience and potential recovery of the communicatively impaired, are not yet clear. There are specific areas that need to be examined more closely. For example, knowledge about a client's self-esteem in relation to communication disability may enhance our understanding of client need and indicate ways to manage a condition more usefully. The role of self-esteem in individual or group therapy and how this determines outcome is an extremely important area to explore in the future. Furthermore, knowledge about self-esteem over time in the trajectory following onset of aphasia could guide clinical decision-making. Bakheit, Barrett and Wood (2004) were able to study 40 acute patients with aphasia in order to look at the relationship between aphasia and self-esteem and to establish whether severity of aphasia correlates significantly with level of self-esteem over time. Measures used were the Western Aphasia Battery (Kertesz, 1982) and the Visual Analogue Self-esteem Scale (Brumfitt and Sheeran, 1999a). Although no significant relationship was found between severity of aphasia and level of self-esteem during the first 6 months of recovery, this study does highlight the complexities in this area. The severity of the aphasia may not have been the most important dimension with which to compare levels of self-esteem. The basis for understanding subjective well-being is that individuals will have entirely idiosyncratic responses to situations, and some aphasic speakers, for example, who may only be mildly impaired may experience distress about this in a way that is not reflected in a more severely impaired speaker. That is, it is the changes to the individual trajectory that may give us meaningful understanding about self-esteem over time, rather than severity of the condition.

Andersson and Fridlund (2002) discuss the life experience of an aphasic person through qualitative analysis of interviews. According to their data, two distinct areas emerged—'interaction' and 'support'. Interaction was perceived as being influenced by feelings of security, such as when the listener waited for the individual to try to communicate, and obstruction experienced from listeners who were not patient and were not prepared to allow the speaker time to communicate. Andersson and Fridland (2002) interpret this as positive and negative experiences of speaking, which have a direct effect on self-esteem. When unhelpful support was given, the individual experience was one of dejection and loss of self-esteem: 'I feel very small, so to speak . . . don't know how to explain it, but . . . When I can't get it out, what I want . . . I feel extremely unhappy' (p. 289).

This aspect of failing to manage a conversation has a resonance in the original work by Harter (1993) on the components of self-esteem. That is, level of self-esteem is determined by the direct experience of competency in communication, which the individual uses to make judgements about self, in combination with the use of social feedback from others. Andersson and Fridland (2002) refer to the experience of failure in conversations causing mistrust of one's ability to interact with others and thus reflecting a feeling of lack of competence.

## Case studies

Case studies 4.1 and 4.2 describe examples of using self-esteem scores in the context of communication impairment.

---

**Case Study 4.1  A young woman with aphasia**

Kathryn was 25 years old when she had an aneurysm. Surgery was completed but she was left with a hemiplegia and aphasia. Prior to this she had lived independently from her parents, in the same town; and had been working as a groom at a horse riding stable but also competed in riding events. In the early stages post-surgery her mood was extremely low. She was reluctant to try to talk to people because of embarrassment. When asked how she generally felt, she took her finger and ran it across her throat indicating that she wanted to die. At 3 months post-surgery, her VASES score was 18/50; revealing an extremely negative view of herself, thus indicating that she could be depressed and needed further investigations. Her scores are shown in Box 4.1.

**Box 4.1   Kathryn 3 months post-surgery: first assessment VASES**

| | |
|---|---|
| Not being understood–being understood | 2 |
| Not confident–confident | 3 |
| Cheerful–not cheerful | 1 |
| Outgoing–not outgoing | 3 |
| Mixed up–not mixed up | 3 |
| Intelligent–not intelligent | 1 |
| Angry–not angry | 1 |
| Trapped–not trapped | 1 |
| Not optimistic–optimistic | 1 |
| Frustrated–not frustrated | 2 |

The speech and language therapist alerted the multidisciplinary team to this result and Kathryn was immediately followed up by the clinical psychologist. She was given antidepressant medication and offered individual and group therapy by the clinical psychologist. She continued with speech and language therapy. In the longer term, after 1 year post-surgery, her VASES score showed some improvement with a score of 36/50 (Box 4.2), and she had begun to regain some skills to improve her quality of life. She had begun to drive again, had returned to the stables to work 1 day a week and had remained in touch with several patients whom she had met in rehabilitation. These people had spontaneously come together and were able to keep in touch, meeting up regularly for support. They had become interested in cooking for each other and regularly held small parties where they would share their interest in cooking (something Kathryn had rarely been interested in pre-surgery).

### Box 4.2    Kathryn, 1 year post-surgery: VASES assessment

| | |
|---|---|
| Not being understood–being understood | 4 |
| Not confident–confident | 3 |
| Cheerful–not cheerful | 4 |
| Outgoing–not outgoing | 3 |
| Mixed up–not mixed up | 4 |
| Intelligent–not intelligent | 3 |
| Angry–not angry | 3 |
| Trapped–not trapped | 4 |
| Not optimistic–optimistic | 4 |
| Frustrated–not frustrated | 4 |

Importantly, through the recovery period and the opportunities for therapy, Kathryn had been able to move towards a more positive evaluation of herself. This came about through a combination of factors. The evidence she gained from her physical recovery allowed her to be able to see herself in a more positive light. Now she could do activities that she had previously thought impossible. Her strongly felt anger in the initial stages had started to reduce, as she was able to regain some of her previous lifestyle. She could see that there was hope for her and she could see that there was still opportunity for improvement. Although there is no evidence of what her VASES score would have been prior to the surgery, it is clear that her self-evaluation was a comparison, strongly linked into her memory of what she had been before the surgery. It was important to ensure that all of her efforts in the recovery phase were not aimed exclusively at regaining the skills she had lost because this would be a risk to her overall well-being. It was essential that Kathryn could evaluate herself in the light of other capabilities so that her focus was not exclusively on the past self. This was protective of her. If Kathryn failed in the future to recover all of her riding skills for example, a reconsideration of her future would be necessary, and that could involve developing new skills that could give her the same sense of well-being. The support and friendship with other rehabilitation patients was able to play a role in developing a new aspect of herself.

---

### Case Study 4.2 A man with severe aphasia

Derek was 61 years old and had worked as a plumber with his own business. He was married and had adult children. Following a major left-sided cerebrovascular accident (CVA) 2 years previously he was left with a right hemiplegia and significant dysphasia. His rehabilitation from the NHS had recently ceased but he still took advantage of a charity support group to mix socially with other people who had had a stroke. At face value, Derek was very cheerful and made full use of his reduced communication skills, attempting to use gesture and facial expression if he could not produce language. The accuracy in gesture use was sometimes in question, but he was always motivated to try to communicate. His wife reported that this was typical of his personality prior to the CVA.

When the VASES was given to Derek he responded to all the items and the final score was 38 (Box 4.3). This was quite a high score considering the extent of his disability, and indicated that he saw himself as confident, cheerful, outgoing, not trapped, and not frustrated in varying degrees. He gave the lowest ratings to 'not being understood' and 'not intelligent', 'not mixed up' and 'angry'.

## Box 4.3 Derek's assessment using the VASES

| | |
|---|---|
| Not being understood–being understood | 3 |
| Not confident–confident | 5 |
| Cheerful–not cheerful | 5 |
| Outgoing–not outgoing | 5 |
| Mixed up–not mixed up | 4 |
| Intelligent–not intelligent | 3 |
| Angry–not angry | 2 |
| Trapped–not trapped | 4 |
| Not optimistic–optimistic | 3 |
| Frustrated–not frustrated | 4 |

Concern was expressed about the amount of anger that Derek had rated on the scale. This had not been evident in his everyday dealings with the therapists and hospital staff. His feeling of anger was the lowest rating on the scale and it posed the question about whether Derek was hiding some of his strong feelings about his situation.

Based on the result, the therapist decided to use a session to try to talk with Derek about his feelings of anger. She began by going over the scale with him and asked him specifically about the rating of '2' on the anger dimension. At this point Derek could have indicated that he had made a mistake or else he could have confirmed his feelings. On looking again at the scale he confirmed his feelings of intense anger. He demonstrated this by banging on the table and becoming very emotional. The therapist was able to ask about what aspects of his situation made him most angry and did this by asking very direct questions in order to facilitate Derek's communication. For example; 'Do you feel angry because you cannot work?' Although this approach is not generally used, there has to be modifications to questioning approaches with someone who has aphasia. For example, the direct closed question may be easier for comprehension and expression rather than the more typical open question that requires the individual to generate self descriptions (e.g. 'Can you tell me about how you are feeling?').

After the session that focused on discussing feelings, Derek appeared to be relieved. The therapist suggested that he consider an appointment with a clinical psychologist. Derek agreed to this and attended. The speech and language therapist gave the clinical psychologist advice about techniques for communicating with Derek. After one appointment Derek was able to state that he was happy to manage without further support.

An important aspect of this case study is the role of the VASES in drawing out views and feelings of an individual that may not have been previously noted. This offers professionals better opportunities to develop appropriate care plans and help the individual to cope more satisfactorily.

---

## Intervention for self-esteem in acquired communication impairments

Little has been reported in the communication impairment literature on interventions that have focused exclusively on improving self-esteem. More commonly, the literature reports an intervention where self-esteem has been one of the outcome measures. Brumfitt and Sheeran (1997) evaluated group therapy for people with aphasia over 10 90-minute sessions. The therapy programme consisted of group communication activities such as sharing personal experiences, videotaping role play activities with discussion, and the use of practical assignments outside the group for evaluation within the group at a later stage. Before the intervention, self-esteem (as measured by the Rosenberg Self-esteem Scale) and communicative competence (as measured by the Functional Communication Profile; Sarno, 1975) were highly correlated ($r = 0.736$, $p < 0.05$). By the end of the therapy sessions, the correlation between self-esteem and communicative competence was much smaller and not significant ($r = 0.422$, $p < 0.01$). This result indicates that communicative function was not related to feelings of self-worth by the end of the intervention. Although a small study of a small group of participants, the separation of communicative competence from self-esteem has important implications for understanding. If it is possible to help an individual gain more self-worth in spite of whether their communication improves, it would be possible to examine methods that focus exclusively on enhancement of self-esteem.

Cunningham and Ward (2003) evaluated an intervention created to train a friend or relative to communicate more effectively with an aphasic speaker. This intervention was evaluated in terms of effects upon communication and on well-being. Positive individual changes and positive trends were found, including improvement in self-esteem as measured by the VASES (Brumfitt and Sheeran, 1999a) when the time within each assessment phase was compared across the pre- and post-intervention phases for the aphasic speakers and their carers.

Ross, Winslow, Marchant and Brumfitt (2006) looked at group intervention involving a social model approach in terms of communication, life participation and psychological well-being for seven people with long-term aphasic difficulties. Measures were taken at a pre-, post- and 3-month follow-up treatment design. The measures used were: Conversational Analysis Profile for People with Aphasia (CAPPA; Whitworth, Perkins and Lesser, 1997) part A, conversation abilities; and CAPPA B, conversation experiences. Psychological well-being was assessed with the Hospital Anxiety and Depression Scale (Zigmond and Snaith, 1983) and the VASES (Brumfitt and Sheeran, 1997). The intervention focused on enabling participants to develop total communication and conversation skills, gain an understanding of disability and rights, and engage in social participation. Thus, none of the intervention was specifically aimed at changing self-esteem. The results, in the form of group means, did not show a statistically significant change in the self-esteem measures over time. The mean increase from pre-intervention to follow-up scores is small and statistically significant (0.3, SD = 5.7, 95% $t$-confidence interval: $-5.0$ to 5.5). However, as the authors note, some gains from the intervention in terms of self-esteem were found. Firstly, each participant was able to understand and respond to the VASES, which confirmed the findings of other studies that have successfully used the assessment with different levels of aphasic speaker (Winslow and Ross, 2006). Four participants showed a sustained increase in self-esteem over time, although three participants showed an overall reduction over time. Ross, Winslow, Marchant and Brumfitt (2006) consider the possibility that the intervention itself may increase insight, which may make the participant become more aware of the challenges to be faced by having a communication impairment. Whether interventions can cause self-esteem to become more negative because of the increased insight is a very interesting possibility, which needs much more investigation.

## Conclusions

It may be the case that evaluation of, and intervention for, impairments associated with self-esteem fit the scope of practice for psychologists more easily than other health professionals. But matters to do with self-esteem may arise during the course of many clinical interactions, whether this is a physiotherapy session, a general case history being taken or language-based therapy interventions in the speech and language therapy context. The professional may start to be concerned that the individual's self-esteem is creating a barrier to progress in any type of health interaction. Individuals may view themselves so negatively that they may feel unable to respond positively to the practice activities that they are being asked to do. For example, in the context of speech and language therapy the individual might be asked to undertake some conversations with one or two strangers as a means of practising specific skills. Low self-esteem is likely to influence the individual's capacity to undertake this type of task as it may feel too challenging. In this situation there is a strong argument for directing the focus of therapy towards enhancing self-worth before the communication task can be successfully completed.

The evidence in this chapter has shown that evaluating self-esteem and working out strategies for helping individuals to raise their self-esteem is in a stage of development for these populations. More methods for evaluating self-esteem are needed, as are therapy programmes that are relevant. It may also be necessary for research to look at subcomponents of self-esteem and whether self-esteem in relation to communication competence exists independently of other aspects of self-esteem. Methods for working on self-esteem need to be examined with reference to other therapeutic approaches occurring alongside and the effectiveness determined. In particular, the progress of self-esteem levels over time during the course of an illness or the course of recovery needs to be further documented.

## References

Andersson S, Fridlund B. The aphasic person's views of the encounter with other people: a grounded theory analysis. J Psychiatr Mental Health Nurs 2002;9:285–292.

Bakheit AMO, Barrett L, Wood J. The relationship between post stroke aphasia and state self esteem. Aphasiology 2004;18:759–764.

Bennett HE, Thomas SA, Austen R, Morris AMS, Lincoln NB. Validation of screening measures for assessing mood in stroke patients. Brit J Clin Psychol 2006;45:367–376.

Blascovich J, Tomaka J. Measures of Self Esteem. Measures of Personality and Social Psychological Attitudes. Academic Press, 1991.

Bowling A. Research Methods in Health. Buckingham: Open University Press, 1997.

Brumfitt SM. The use of repertory grids with aphasic people. In: Beail N (ed.) Repertory Grid Technique and Personal Constructs. Croom Helm, 1985; pp. 89–106.

Brumfitt SM. Losing your sense of self: what aphasia can do. Clinical Forum Aphasiology 1993;7:569–591.

Brumfitt SM. Psychosocial aspects of aphasia: Speech and language therapists' views on professional practice. Disabil Rehabil 2006;28:523–534.

Brumfitt SM, Sheeran P. Group therapy for aphasic people. Disabil Rehabil 1997;19:221–231.

Brumfitt SM, Sheeran P. The Visual Analogue Self Esteem Scale. Bicester, UK: Winslow Press, 1999a.

Brumfitt SM, Sheeran P. The development and validation of the Visual Analogue Self Esteem Scale (VASES). Brit J Clin Psychol 1999b;38:387–400.

Burns RB. The Self Concept. London: Longman, 1979.

Cant R. Rehabilitation following stroke: a participant perspective. Disabil Rehabil 1997;19:297–304.

Chang AM, Mackenzie AE. State Self Esteem following stroke. Stroke 1998;29:2325–2328.

Code C, Helmsley G, Herrman M. The emotional impact of aphasia. Semin Speech Lang 1999;20:19–31.

Cunningham R, Ward C. Evaluation of a training programme to facilitate conversation between people with aphasia and their partners Aphasiology 2003;17:687–707.

Emler N. Self Esteem, the Costs and Causes of Low Self Worth. York: Joseph Rowntree Foundation, 2001.

Festinger L. A theory of social comparison processes. Human Relations 1954;7:117–140.

Gainotti G. Emotional, psychological and psychosocial impairments of aphasic patients: an introduction. Aphasiology 1997;11:635–650.

Gray-Little B, Hafdahl A. Factors influencing racial comparisons of self esteem: a quantitative review. Psychol Bull 2000;126:26–54.

Harter S. Causes and consequences of low self esteem in children and adolescents. In: Baumeister RF (ed.) Self Esteem: the Puzzle of Low Self Regard. New York: Plenum, 1993.

Heatherton TF, Polivy J. Development and validation of a scale for measuring state self esteem. J Pers Soc Psychol 1991;60:895–910.

Hoffman T, Worrall L. Designing effective written health education materials: considerations for health professionals. Disabil Rehabil 2004;26:1166–1173.

Houts PS, Doak CC, Doak L, Loscalzo MJ. The role of pictures in improving health communication: A review of research on attention, comprehension, recall and adherence. Patient Educ Couns 2006;61:173–190.

Jerome AC, Fujiki M, Brinton B, James SL. Self-esteem in children with specific language impairment. J Speech Lang Hear Res 2002;45:700–714.

Josephs RA, Bosson JK, Jacobs CG. Self esteem maintenance processes: why low self esteem may be resistant to change. Pers Soc Psychol Bull 2003;29:920–933.

Katz A. Leading Lads. London: Topman, 2000.

Kertesz A. Western Aphasia Battery. London: Harcourt, Brace and Jovanovich, 1982.

Krause N, Alexander G. Self esteem and psychological distress in later life. J Aging Health 1990;2:419–438.

Letourneau PY. The psychological effects of aphasia. In: Lafond D, DeGiovani R, Joanette Y, Ponzio J, Taylor Sarno M (eds) Living with Aphasia. San Diego, CA: Singular Publishing, 1993.

Manuel JC, Balkrishnan R, Camacho F, Paterson Smith B, Koman LA. Factors associated with self esteem in pre adolescents and adolescents with cerebral palsy. J Adolesc Health 2003;32:456–458.

Marmot M. Self esteem and health. BMJ 2003;327:57–575.

McAndrew E. The relationship between self esteem and language disordered children. Child Lang Teaching Ther 1999;15:219–232.

Muller D. Managing psychosocial adjustment to aphasia. Semin Speech Lang 1999;20:85–92.

Pound C, Parr S, Woolf C. Beyond Aphasia. Bicester: Speechmark, 2000.

Rees CE, Ford JE, Sheard CE. Patient information leaflets for prostate cancer: which leaflets should health professionals recommend? Patient Educ Couns 2003;49:263–272.

Rhodes N, Wood W. Self esteem and intelligence affect influencibility, the mediating role of message reception. Psychol Bull 1992;111:156–71.

Rose T, Worrall L, McKenna KT. The effectiveness of aphasia friendly principles for printed health education materials for people with aphasia following stroke. Aphasiology 2003;17:947–963.

Rosenberg M. Society and the Adolescent Self Image. Princeton: Princeton University Press, 1965.

Ross A, Winslow I, Marchant P, Brumfitt SM. Evaluation of communication, life participation and psychological well being in chronic aphasia: the influence of group intervention. Aphasiology 2006;20:427–448.

Santrock JW. Adolescence. New York: McGraw-Hill, 2001.

Sarno MT. The Functional Communication Profile: Manual of Directions. Rehabilitation Monographs 1975;42:1–32.

Sorgaard KW, Heikkila J, Hansson L, Vinding H, Bjarnason O, Bengtson-Tops A, Merinder L, Nilsson L, Sandlund M, Middleboe T. Self esteem in persons with schizophrenia. A Nordic multicentre study. J Mental Health 2002;11:405–415.

Starkstein SE, Robinson RG. Aphasia and depression. Aphasiology 1988;2:1–20.

Tennen H, Affleck G. The puzzles of self esteem, a clinical perspective. In: Baumeister R (ed.) Self Esteem, the Puzzle of Low Self Regard. New York: Plenum, 1993.

Tesser A. Advanced Social Psychology. McGraw-Hill, 1995.

Townend E, Brady M, McLaughlan K. A systematic evaluation of the adaptation of depression diagnostic methods for stroke survivors who have aphasia. Stroke 2007;38:3076–3083.

Vickery C. Assessment and correlates of self esteem following stroke using a pictorial measure. Clin Rehabil 2006;20:1075–1084.

Vickery C, Sepehri A, Evans CC. Self esteem in an acute stroke rehabilitation sample: a control group comparison. Clin Rehabil 2008;22:179–187.

Westbrook LE, Bauman LJ, Shinnar S. Applying stigma theory to epilepsy: a test of a conceptual model. J Pediatr Psychol 1992;17:633–649.

Whelan A, Haywood P, Galloway S. Low self esteem: group cognitive behavioural therapy. Brit J Learning Disabilities 2007;35:125–130.

Whitworth A, Perkins L, Lesser R. Conversational Analysis Profile for People with Aphasia. London: Whurr Publishers, 1997.

Winslow I, Ross A. An evaluation of the effectiveness of a multiagency partnership provision of groups for people with aphasia. Evidence based practice: a challenge for speech and language therapists. Proceedings of the CPLOL Conference 5–7 September 2006 (www.cplol.org).

Yesavage JA, Brink TL, Rose TL, Lum O, Huang V, Adey M, Leirer VO. Development and validation of a geriatric depression screening scale: a preliminary report. J Psychiatr Res 1983;17:37–40.

Yovetich WMS, Leschied AW, Flicht J. Self esteem of school aged children who stutter. J Fluency Dis 2000;25:143–153.

Zigmond AS, Snaith RP. The Hospital Anxiety and Depression Scale. Acta Psychiatr Scand 1983;67:361–370.

Zung W, Richards C, Gables C, Short M. Self rating depression scale in an outpatient clinic Arch Gen Psychiat 1965;13:508–515.

# 5 The Role of Well-Being in Quality of Life for the Person with Acquired Communication Impairments

**Madeline Cruice**

Well-being is an important consideration for any professional (clinician or researcher) working with people who have acquired communication difficulties. The role of well-being in clients' lives and its relevance to professionals depends largely on how the term 'well-being' has been interpreted. This chapter explores well-being as one conceptualisation of quality of life, alongside its mainstream partner, health-related quality of life. Emphasis is placed on understanding the differences amongst the components of subjective well-being, as well as the difference between subjective and psychological well-being. The chapter refers to the general literature on quality of life, in addition to well-being and health-related quality of life literature in stroke, spinal cord injury and ageing populations. Within speech and language therapy, the most frequently investigated clinical population, aphasia is discussed in detail, and new research in dysarthria is also briefly illustrated. The chapter reviews a range of instruments that may be considered appropriate for evaluating clients' well-being, and concludes by alerting readers to measurement concerns in this field. Throughout the chapter, three real cases of people with aphasia taken from the author's own research are used to illustrate the concepts and relationships raised in this chapter.

## An introduction to the relevant concepts and terminology

Quality of life (QoL) is an exponentially developing field, with new measurement instruments being designed every month. Possibly because of this rapid explosion of interest in the field, there is no real consensus on how QoL is defined, and what it comprises. Definitions can reflect the preoccupations of the particular discipline (derived from the different nature of care and experiences that the professional has with the patient), different exposure to QoL measures, or the agenda of the institution that is defining QoL (McKevitt, Redfern, La-Placa and Wolfe, 2003). For example, physiotherapy defines QoL in terms of mobility and independence, and nursing palliative care staff refer to QoL as freedom from pain (Bearon, 1988), whilst physiotherapists and occupational therapists refer more to social aspects and physical function when defining QoL for patients than do physicians (McKevitt *et al*, 2003). The gold standard of definitions is perceived as that defined by the World Health Organization as:

> an individual's perception of their position in life in the context of the culture and value systems in which they live and in relation to their goals, expectations, standards and concerns
>
> *(World Health Organization, 1993. p. 5)*

A small-scale alternative quality of life group, this time in Canada, defines QoL as:

> 'the degree to which a person enjoys the important possibilities of his or her life. Possibilities result from the opportunities and limitations each person has in his/her life and reflect the interaction of personal and environmental factors. Enjoyment has two components: the experience of satisfaction or the possession or achievement of some characteristic'
>
> *(University of Toronto, Centre of Health Promotion;*
> *http://www.utoronto.ca/qol/concepts.htm, accessed on 12 March 2007)*

Other definitions of QoL are more simplistic, listing the factors that give quality in life such as happy marriages, contentment, social relations, income, standards of living, and possession of goods (Seed and Lloyd, 1997). However one chooses to define QoL, the dichotomy of internal and external, objective and subjective, and health and well-being, are universally accepted concepts.

Quality of life is widely agreed as a dichotomy of internal (or private) and external (or public). Baldwin, Godfrey and Propper (1990) describe it as the quality of an individual's life that is private and is a reflection on how well his or her life is going; and the quality of the living conditions around an individual, which are independent of how well the individual's own life goes. The internal includes an individual's values and beliefs, desires and goals, personality attributes, coping strategies, and spiritual status; the external includes both the natural environment, such as weather and air quality, as well as the societal environment of institutions, schools, services, government, community and safety (Spilker and Revicki, 1996). George and Bearon (1980) conceptualise it as the experience of life, and the conditions of life. The *experience* of life is subjective, measured using instruments of life satisfaction and self-esteem. The *conditions* of life are objective, measured using instruments of general health and functional status, and socioeconomic status. QoL is also seen as the degree of fit that exists between the perception of an objective situation (external) and the person's needs or aspirations (internal), which is largely how we make our judgements of QoL. This degree of fit can also be described as the congruence between a person's aspirations and their accomplishments, as perceived by the person involved (Tate, Dijkers and Johnson-Greene, 1996).

The objective-subjective dichotomy is also widely understood in QoL. Objective QoL components are physical health, functional health, cognitive functioning, the existence of a social network, economic status and environmental factors, whereas subjective QoL components comprise health perceptions, life satisfaction, self-esteem and sense of control (Birren and Dieckmann in Birren, Lubben, Cichowlas Rowe and Deutchman, 1991). Objective and subjective components are typically distinct from one another, and complement each other to give an *overall* QoL. More recently, QoL components are assessed from both perspectives, for example, counting the number of social contacts in an individual's social network (objective) and assessing the level of support the individual derives from the social network (subjective). Personal values are also important in QoL, and are needed to make sense of either objective or subjective evaluations (see Cummins in Felce and Perry, 1995). For example, the size of someone's income (objective) may contribute little to the quality of life for a person whose values are non-materialist (value), although satisfaction with income (subjective, i.e. ability to meet needs) might still carry high weight.

### The relationships between health, well-being and quality of life

Quality of life is an overarching umbrella construct and includes both health and well-being. In the last 50 years, these two conceptual approaches to QoL measurement have evolved to different degrees (Kaplan and Anderson, 1996). The first, health-related quality of life (HRQoL), grows from the tradition of health status measurements, guided by the World Health Organization's definition of health. It is a much stronger conceptual approach than well-being, and is embedded in the majority of QoL instruments that exist. It has influenced the field so much that when someone is asked about their QoL, they automatically think of their health. Yet clinicians and people who are chronically ill or disabled know that there is more to QoL than health. The second conceptual approach is based on the notion that QoL is something independent of health status, and relates to psychological variables, well-being and life satisfaction. The rise of well-being in QoL has been largely due to the increased recognition of the patient's perceptions in healthcare, and the accompanying increasing credit and use of qualitative research methodologies, which are typically employed to investigate this field. Well-being has been referred to, or qualified further, as *personal* well-being, *total* well-being, *subjective* well-being, and *general* well-being, all of which are assumed to mean the same thing (Pope and Tarlov, 1991). The term *subjective well-being* will be used in this chapter.

Under these two approaches of health and well-being, exists a further salient feature in QoL, which is a number of separate domains that collectively constitute total health or total well-being.

In HRQoL, all of the domains relate to health. For example, within the stroke literature, four domains are important and common in assessment (de Haan *et al.*, 1995):

1. *physical health* (disease related symptoms);
2. *functional health* (self-care and physical activity level);
3. *psychological health* (cognitive functioning, emotional status, general perceptions of health, well-being, life satisfaction and happiness;
4. *social health* (social contacts and interactions).

Well-being is rarely explicitly explored in stroke; however, the reader will note that it is included under the banner of *psychological health* above. In well-being, specifically *subjective* well-being, the domains are different constructs, and are not tagged with the suffix of well-being. These domains are explained below. Unfortunately, some researchers have created confusion in the literature by generating well-being domains, referring to them as *physical, mental, social, emotional* and *material* well-being. This represents a misuse of the term well-being.

## Subjective well-being

There is only a small degree of variation in subjective well-being (SWB), and definitions generally reflect the following components (Fuhrer, 1994):

1. it is an individual's global judgement of their life experience;
2. judgements are made along a continuum that ranges from positive to negative;
3. it reflects the individual's implicit standards;
4. it involves both a cognitive and emotionally toned judgement.

The consensus is that SWB comprises three different constructs of life satisfaction, positive affect and negative affect. While it can be argued that life satisfaction and affect are indeed only two constructs, it is important to recognise that positive and negative affect are different concepts, i.e. the absence of negative affect does not equal positive affect. These constructs are described in further detail below:

- *Life satisfaction*: is an evaluation of the overall condition of one's existence through a comparison of one's aspirations and one's achievements (George and Bearon, 1980). This is essentially a global cognitively based evaluation (George, 1981; Menhert, Krauss, Nadler and Boyd, 1990). It involves feelings about the past (McDowell and Newell, 1996), and has an enduring long-term quality (Ryff, 1989).

- *Positive affect*: is the experience of positive feelings, such as joy, pleasure and elation (Menhert, Krauss, Nadler and Boyd, 1990), and is more dependent on external stimulation than internal control (Birren, Lubben, Cichowlas Rowe and Deutchman, 1991). It is sometimes referred to as happiness, which is the shorter-term, transitory feelings of well-being in response to day-to-day events (George, 1981; Horley in Tate, Dijkers and Johnson-Greene, 1996). Ryff (1989) states that happiness can be operationalised as the balance between positive and negative affect.
- *Negative affect*: is the experience of negative feelings, such as anxiety or sadness (Menhert, Krauss, Nadler and Boyd, 1990), and is more dependent on internal control than external stimulation (Birren, Lubben, Cichowlas Rowe and Deutchman, 1991). It can be operationalised as the absence of distress.

Morale is sometimes considered important in discussions of SWB (Fuhrer, 1994), and is described as: willingness to endure hardship (Fuhrer, 1994); optimism for the future (McDowell and Newell, 1996); feelings of social cohesion, motivation and commitment to group goals (George, 1981); and a person's mental orientation, enthusiasm, confidence, sadness or depression (Tate, Dijkers and Johnson-Greene, 1996). It is perceived as longer term than happiness.

Psychological well-being (PWB) is typically indicated by mental health, cognitive judgements of overall life satisfaction, and positive and negative emotions (both of which can be expressed as states or traits) (Birren, Lubben, Cichowlas Rowe and Deutchman, 1991). Negative emotions are most commonly considered to be anxiety and depression. As such, it is a combination of SWB and mental health. PWB is also thought to include coping skills, self-esteem and adjustment to illness (Fallowfield, 1990; Tate, Dijkers and Johnson-Greene, 1996). According to Carol Ryff, a well-known researcher in the field, PWB also includes positive relations with others, autonomy, purpose in life and personal growth (Ryff, 1989). Her measurement instrument appears to tap all of the said components, and is organised into six dimensions of PWB. Versions of her instrument have been used as an outcome measure in aphasia research and are referred to later in this chapter.

## Well-being in communication-impaired populations

The majority of research into well-being has been carried out among people with aphasia. Qualitative research reveals that mental attitudes, sense of self, autonomy and choice, and emotions are important to the lives of people with aphasia and their relatives (Le Dorze and Brassard, 1995;

Hoen, Thelander and Worsley, 1997; Zemva, 1999). Quantitative research has investigated psychosocial functioning and adjustment, subjective and psychological well-being, life satisfaction and other subjective constructs of people with aphasia (Hemsley and Code, 1996; Lyon *et al.*, 1997; Records and Baldwin, 1996; Hoen, Thelander and Worsley, 1997; Sarno, 1997; Engell, Huber and Hütter, 1998; Hinckley, 1998; Hilari and Byng, 2001; Cruice, Worrall, Hickson and Murison, 2003; Ross and Wertz, 2003). The limited number of studies that *specifically* discuss psychological well-being and life satisfaction in aphasia is elaborated on first, and then new research into the emotional, social and psychological changes with dysarthria is outlined.

## Well-being in aphasia

There is a proven link between language, communication and psychological well-being in older Australian men and women with mild to moderate chronic aphasia (Cruice, Worrall, Hickson and Murison, 2003). This study of 30 participants used the condensed version of the Ryff short-form Psychological Well-being scale as devised by Hoen, Thelander and Worsley (1997), and traditional speech and language therapy assessments: the Western Aphasia Battery (Kertesz, 1982) and the Communication Activities of Daily Living Revised (CADL-2: Holland, Frattali and Fromm, 1999). The research found that participants with better language and better functional communication abilities had significantly higher psychological well-being. Three of the six PWB subscales were statistically significant: *'personal growth'* (being open to new experiences), *'positive relations with others'* (having satisfying high quality relationships), and *'self acceptance'* (a positive attitude towards oneself and one's past life). These relationships are illustrated well in Case studies 5.1 to 5.3, using Henry, Jane and Florence (pseudonyms), who were drawn from the research sample of 30 participants. It is important to note that in the overall QoL field, a population size ($N$) of 30 is considered small-scale research. This is because many QoL studies typically utilise unit- or hospital-wide methods of data collection, yielding participants in the hundreds. Case data also include measures of emotional state using the Geriatric Depression Scale (GDS, 15-item version: Sheikh and Yesavage, 1986); individuals' engagement in communication activities and social activities, which was self-reported using checklists; and their social network, which was recorded as the number of important people in individuals' lives. Table 5.1 details the numerical scores or qualitative options for each of the measures per case.

Case studies 5.1 to 5.3 describe the language, communication and psychological well-being status in three individuals from the study of older Australian men and women with mild to moderate chronic aphasia conducted by Cruice, Worrall, Hickson and Murison (2003).

**Table 5.1** Case information: language functioning, communication ability and activities, social activities and network, emotional state, overall quality of life, and psychological well-being.

| Areas of evaluation | Henry | Jane | Florence |
|---|---|---|---|
| Western Aphasia Battery Quotient | 64.4 | 78 | 87.8 |
| Spontaneous Speech | 15 | 17 | 20 |
| Comprehension | 7.2 | 7.5 | 9 |
| Repetition | 3.4 | 7.4 | 6.6 |
| Naming | 6.6 | 7.1 | 8.3 |
| CADL-2 Score (max. = 100) | 56 | 84 | 71 |
| Number of communicative activities (max. = 45) | 23 | 35 | 30 |
| Number of social activities (max. = 20) | 13 | 15 | 15 |
| Response to social activities | Would like to be doing more | Would like to be doing more | Satisfied |
| Number of people in social network | 11 | 23 | 28 |
| GDS score (upwards of 5 = depressive symptoms) | 12 | 1 | 0 |
| Overall quality of life rating | Very poor | Average | Very good |
| Psychological well-being total score (max. = 120) | 64 | 75 | 106 |
| Autonomy subscale (max. = 20) | 9 | 10 | 15 |
| Environmental mastery subscale (max. = 20) | 5 | 11 | 17 |
| Personal growth subscale (max. = 20) | 16 | 15 | 19 |
| Positive relations with the others subscale (max. = 20) | 13 | 12 | 19 |
| Purpose in life subscale (max. = 20) | 12 | 15 | 18 |
| Self-acceptance subscale (max. = 20) | 9 | 12 | 18 |

### Case Study 5.1 Henry

Henry was a 77-year-old retired police officer, living with his wife in their own home. He'd had a stroke 4 years ago (48 months), had a moderate to mild aphasic linguistic impairment, but moderate functional communication ability. Henry's self-report on the GDS suggested moderately severe depressive symptoms, and he rated his overall QoL as *very poor* (minimum point on the scale).

### Case Study 5.2 Jane

Jane was a single, 64-year-old retired TAB (betting agency) supervisor, who lived independently in her own villa within a retirement village complex. Jane had a stroke 65 months prior to the study, had mild aphasic linguistic impairment, and was a particularly effective communicator as evidenced by her reasonably high CADL-2 score. Jane's self-report on the GDS suggested normal emotional state, and she rated her overall QoL as *average* (mid-point on the scale).

---

### Case Study 5.3 Florence

Florence was a widowed, 72-year-old retired corner-store owner, who now lived with her family in the large family home. Florence had a stroke just less than 2 years ago (23 months) and had a very mild aphasic linguistic impairment. She rated herself with maximum life quality, *very good*, and scored zero on the GDS, reflecting normal emotional state. Despite her mild impairment, she demonstrated some communication difficulties on daily functional tasks (compare her CADL-2 score with Jane's).

---

Other case studies from the author's larger study have been published (see Cruice, Worrall and Hickson, 2006) and reiterate the importance of well-being in aphasia. That paper reported on the findings of qualitative interviews from four women from the sample, and concluded that: 'perceiving QoL . . . depends on a number of factors that include having positive experiences in sharing one's life with others, being content with one's living arrangement, having independence and control over aspects of one's life, engaging in meaningful and personally rewarding activities (especially leisure), dealing with loss and change, and continuing to grow personally' (p. 23). Unintentionally, these findings reflect the content of the Ryff PWB subscales. Ongoing analysis of the interview findings from all 30 participants suggests that a *positive personal outlook* is important in overall QoL with aphasia (Cruice, Hill, Worrall and Hickson, *in press*). Participants' comments conveyed how they still managed to do things, for example: 'If I take me time, I succeed. I feel capable'; and others reflected a positive attitude of acceptance or defiance towards their personal difficulties, for example: 'It's not what it used to be but you got to accept it' and 'It doesn't worry me, I'll just say bugger ya, I don't care'. Many participants qualified the difficulties they had now with activities, commenting 'but I can do a couple of little things'; 'but I think on this I can cope; but I've got used to that now; so I have to try other things'. Whilst the relationship between positive personal outlook and PWB in aphasia needs further in-depth study, this research presents some interesting preliminary findings.

Psychological well-being, as well as overall QoL, has been studied in a small group of 18 adults with aphasia, and 18 non-brain-injured adults (Ross and Wertz, 2003). The authors chose the non-standardised 11-item Psychological Well-being Index (PWI) by Lyon *et al.* (1997), and the World Health Organization Quality of Life Instrument abbreviated version (WHOQOL-BREF: the WHOQOL Group, 1998) to compare the two groups. The research demonstrated that aphasic adults had significantly lower PWB and overall QoL than the non-brain-injured adults.

Most of the existing literature describes PWB state, and only two studies to date have investigated change in PWB. Hoen, Thelander and Worsley

(1997) reported increased PWB on most subscales for 35 aphasic adults and 12 relatives attending group therapies at an aphasia centre in North York. Van der Gaag *et al.* (2005) reported increased QoL and communication for 38 men and women and 22 of their relatives, who attended a range of group therapies based in a charity organisation in the UK. Although that research does not tap PWB explicitly, their qualitative interviews revealed that participants had increased levels of self-confidence and an increased desire to participate. These improvements were manifested in many aspects of daily life—going out more, going on a holiday for the first time since their stroke, talking to strangers in shops and in the street again, wanting more social contact with friends and family, and feeling better about themselves (Van der Gaag *et al.*, 2005, p. 375). Using the Ryff PWB dimension approach, these changes can be construed as 'positive relations with others' and 'self-acceptance', but also suggest a need to consider communicative confidence or readiness (see Lyon *et al.*, 1997).

### Psychological distress in communication-impaired stroke survivors

A concept that is related to but distinct from PWB is *psychological distress*. New measurement instruments such as the Burden of Stroke Scale (BOSS: Doyle, McNeil, Hula and Mikolic, 2003) and its companion scales of Communication Difficulty (CD) and Communication-Associated Psychological Distress (CAPD) highlight how important psychological distress is to communication-impaired stroke survivors. The BOSS, CD, CAPD and positive and negative mood scales were administered to 135 communication-impaired stroke survivors (mean age 61.5 years, mean months post-onset 61.3 months) and 146 stroke survivors without communication impairments (Doyle, McNeil, Hula and Mikolic, 2003). The research demonstrated that communication-impaired participants had significantly worse CD and CAPD than their counterparts without communication impairments. The study also revealed that linguistic severity and communication difficulty are correlated and possibly predictive of one another, but that linguistic severity and psychological distress are not. Although further research is needed, this study clearly demonstrates future potential by providing the tools for eliciting patient-perceived communication-associated psychological distress.

### Psychosocial issues in dysarthria

Psychosocial issues have been generally very poorly studied in motor speech disorders, until publication of a significant piece of research conducted with dysarthric adults (Walshe, 2002). Part of this research was conducted as interviews with 11 adults with dysarthria (gradual onset caused by progressive diseases) and contributes to the evidence base in dysarthria. The research detailed the emotional changes experienced by dysarthric speakers, including embarrassment and sensitivity; lack of confidence and feeling inadequate; worry and fear; feeling hurt and upset; loss of control (from perceived loss of independence and role change); frustration and annoyance; feeling nervous and uncomfortable; and feeling lonely and isolated. Interviews were also analysed to reveal the following life changes (note that these were not necessarily caused by the dysarthria; e.g. physical disability had more influence on leisure activities than dysarthria for the 11 participants, who all had some form of physical disability): change in role, employment, leisure activities, social life, relationships, self-perception (more self-conscious; less confident, sociable and in control; and inadequate) and communication behaviour (Walshe, 2002). A study of the impact of spasmodic dysphonia on the lives of six adults found similar affective and social role changes to those found by Walshe (2002). Interviewees described feeling embarrassed, frustrated, hopeless, disheartened, self-conscious, and less intelligent, confident and competent (Baylor, Yorkston and Eadie, 2005), as well as quitting employment, avoiding changing or new employment, and giving up community and social activities.

One of the major findings of Walshe's work was that the majority of participants perceived their physical disability to be more important than their speech, and this serves as a reminder to speech and language therapists to consider communication within the context of other abilities and disabilities. Participants also felt that family, friends and others avoided talking with them or ignored them and the dysarthria, and perceived these communication partners as impatient and embarrassed by the person's speech. Participants also commonly referred to the feeling of being evaluated by the communication partner, being more self-conscious when speaking, and watching for communication partner's reactions, which they described as predominantly negative (Walshe, 2002).

The research also explored changes in communication behaviours with dysarthria, which are included here in the chapter because of their impact on social situations. Findings illustrated that participants changed their communication style, avoided normal everyday communication situations (such as asking for items in shops and using the telephone), avoided words, and changed their stance in communicative interactions, that is, they listened rather than took part in a conversation depending on who they were communicating with (Walshe, 2002). Participants described how they used non-verbal communication, kept conversations short, and were unable to make small talk or convey emotion in their voice. These avoidance tactics and reducing involvement in situations and conversations are assumed to be effective coping strategies, but will likely have quite negative consequences on social life participation. Avoidance tactics are not specific to individuals with dysarthria, as spasmodic dysphonia speakers also reported using them (Baylor, Yorkston and Eadie, 2005). In summary, Walshe's study highlights the psychosocial issues for adults with progressive dysarthria and suggests that the emotional, psychological and social issues are shared with aphasic speakers. It paves the way for future research into the experiences of adults with acquired non-progressive dysarthria as well as adults who have developmental dysarthria.

Walshe has published some of her doctoral research to date in a paper on the negative impact of dysarthria on speakers' self-concept (Walshe, 2004). Self-concept was defined as the 'collection of self-knowledge and self-conceptions, formed through personal experiences and interpretation of the environment' and involves 'how we think of ourselves now, how we imagine ourselves in the future and the way we thought about ourselves in the past' (p. 10). The measurement instrument used in this study was the modified version of the Head Injury Semantic Differential Scale (Tyerman and Humphrey, 1984). Four of the 20 items were deemed not applicable for the dysarthric population, and were replaced with new items identified through interviews with dysarthric speakers. The constructs contributing to self-concept are: un-selfconscious, happy, in control, relaxed, satisfied, attractive, hopeful, self-confident, stable, of value, assertive, not irritable, caring, capable, independent, intelligent, competent, sociable, friendly and patient (Walshe, 2004). Participants rate their Present and Past self at the same time.

The study of 31 adults with acquired dysarthria (some participants had progressive prognoses; some had physical impairment) demonstrated that the majority of participants rated their Present Self significantly more negatively than their Past Self on 18 of the 20 constructs (Walshe, 2004). Participants showed no significant change in self on friendly-unfriendly and intelligent-stupid constructs, both of which they rated highly, i.e. positively. Only 2 out of the 31 adults had positive changes in self-concept, i.e. their Present Self scored higher than their Past Self. As well as using the change scores to derive meaning of self-concept, the reader can peruse the averaged ratings for each item, which are reported in Figure 1 of Walshe's paper. Using that information we can identify that the sample of 31 adults rated their Present Self as: caring, capable, intelligent, competent and friendly (5 positive); as well as self-conscious, tense, dissatisfied, unattractive, lacking in confidence, unstable, unassertive, irritable, withdrawn and impatient (10 negative). Five constructs were borderline between positive and negative: happy-unhappy, in control-helpless, hopeful-despondent, of value-worthless and independent-dependent.

The paper reports on three interesting and possibly confounding variables in the data: additional physical impairment, progressive versus non-progressive dysarthrias (and conditions), and the methodological difficulties with reporting on Past Self. With respect to the emphasis of this current chapter, the third variable is the most interesting, as it is dependent on memory, is influenced by cognitive and emotional states, and can become idealised upon reflection, leading to even greater discrepancy in ratings (Walshe, 2004). Nonetheless, the work represents a significant contribution to increasing professionals' understanding of self-concept and psychosocial issues for dysarthric speakers, and should encourage clinicians and researchers to continue developing this knowledge base.

## Variables associated with well-being

A range of variables are associated with well-being. They are either correlates or predictors of well-being, but can also be associated with each other. They include: emotional state; social networks and relationships; social and daily activities; identity; and self-esteem. These are elaborated on below in the aforementioned order.

Research in chronic aphasia has illustrated a significant relationship between emotional state and psychological well-being. An individual's emotional state can be referred to as emotional *health* or emotional *distress*, mood (implied to be short-term), depression (implied to be long-term) and anxiety. The author's study of 30 older men and women demonstrated that participants' better emotional health (fewer depressive symptoms as self-assessed on the GDS) correlated strongly with their higher psychological well-being (total score, as well as self-acceptance, purpose in life and environmental mastery subscales) ranging from $r = -0.6$ to $-0.7$ at $p = 0.005$ significance level (Cruice, 2001). Readers can return to the case data and compare Henry's high GDS score of 12 with Florence's zero GDS score (low GDS scores indicate more desirable states, thus a negative correlation with PWB scores is expected) and their respective PWB scores of 64 and 106. As post-stroke depression can be present in as many as 70% of people with aphasia (Sarno, 1993), and is one of three major issues in post-stroke QoL (Bays, 2001), it is essential for professionals to assess the client's emotional state in any well-being evaluation.

Furthermore, mood has a significant impact on functioning, motivation and subsequent recovery after stroke (Stern, 1999), and 'plays an important role in choice of life goals and determines intensity of goal-striving behaviour' (Nair and Wade, 2003, p. 525). As we have learnt earlier in the chapter that individuals make judgements about their life satisfaction by comparing their aspirations (goals) with their achievements (see page 89), the clinician's role in appropriate goal setting with patients or clients becomes even more important. The greatest challenge often lies in making the goals realistic and achievable. Ozer (1999) suggests that patients need experience in understanding the rate of their own progress, before they are able realistically to predict their functioning in the situation, and subsequently set attainable, appropriate goals. Finally, as stated earlier, an individual's *affective experience* is particularly important in SWB, and includes both the dimension of *positive* affect and the dimension of *negative* affect (Birren, Lubben, Cichowlas Rowe and Deutchman, 1991). Patterns of emotional experiences are influenced by daily events and their relation to life tasks, as well as personal strivings (Oishi, Diener, Suh and Lucas, 1999). The way in which people process both positive and negative experiences and the events associated with them strongly determines people's mental health outcomes (Birren, Lubben, Cichowlas Rowe and Deutchman, 1991).

There is a strong link between social activities and/or relationships and PWB (Fuhrer, 1996). However, the degree of causation or prediction between these two constructs is not clear. Involvement with other people certainly contributes to the life satisfaction of many persons; however, it is equally likely that when people feel positively about their lives, they become more sociable (Fuhrer, 1996). Case data confirm the association between social *relationships* and well-being, but contradict the association between social *activities* and well-being. Henry, Jane and Florence show a trend of increasing size of social network (11 to 23 to 28 social contacts) and increasing PWB; however, the number of their social activities is too similar to create any trend. Instead, the case data suggest that being *satisfied* with the number of social activities may be associated with well-being, and that Henry and Jane, who would like to be doing more social activities, have lower PWB.

A recent study of 1669 older Americans (non-brain-injured) investigated the socialisation patterns of participants, and identified a range of social networks (Fiori, Antonucci and Cortina, 2006). Two of these networks were found to be *restricted*, described as a 'nonfamily network' and a 'nonfriends network'. Fiori and colleagues found that 'depressive symptomatology was highest for individuals in the nonfriends network and lowest for individuals in the diverse network' (p. 25). Simply stated, it seemed that having friends but not family was better than having family but not friends. This research continues to confirm the strong link between depression and limited socialisation that is already known to exist, and more specifically identifies the importance of friends in social networks. A similar feature is noted in the case data. Henry, who rated himself with moderately severe depressive symptoms, is certainly more limited in his social contacts than Jane or Florence. He is, however, by no means socially isolated with 11 social contacts. Based on the larger study of 30 participants, older adults with aphasia had significantly fewer social contacts than similarly aged non-brain-injured older adults, with fewer friends present in their networks (Cruice, Worrall and Hickson, ).

Oishi, Diener, Suh and Lucas (1999) also confirm the association between activities and well-being, stating that *daily* well-being can be predicted from the degree of autonomy and competence in activities. They move forwards the discussion of the role of activities in well-being, suggesting that people gain a sense of satisfaction out of activities that are congruent with their values. Activities that reflect intrinsic needs, such as personal growth and relationships, are more satisfying that activities that reflect extrinsic needs, such as social recognition and physical attractiveness (Oishi, Diener, Suh and Lucas, 1999).

Changing activities is also linked to well-being, particularly in older persons. In the literature on ageing, changing one's activities is often described as one of several processes that enable the older person to retain a sense of self-esteem in the face of declining functioning. Here the work of Brandstadter and Greve (see Lundh and Nolan, 1996) is relevant. They describe three processes called assimilation, accommodation and immunisation. In ageing, it is accommodation processes that explain a good subjective QoL (Lundh and Nolan, 1996). Accommodation involves replacing current activities, goals and aspirations with equally valued new ones. These researchers also found that it is the *meaning* and the *significance* of the activity to the person, and not the *nature* of the activity, that is more important. As the case data possibly suggest, *satisfaction* with activities may be important. Professionals could apply these processes to the adult acquired neurogenic field to explore why patients and clients take part in activities, how and why patients or clients change their activities, and what the impact on their well-being may be. It would also be worthwhile to reflect on what the professional's role is in goal and aspiration setting with adults with communication impairments.

Recently *Topics in Stroke Rehabilitation* produced a special issue (volume 13, issue 1, 2006) dedicated to living successfully with stroke and aphasia, and nearly all of the papers touched on aspects of well-being in the lives of people with aphasia. In particular, Hinckley (2006) reviewed 20 documents written by people with aphasia to answer 'what does it take to live successfully with stroke and aphasia?' and found four main themes emerging. Two related specifically to well-being, namely, adapting one's perception of oneself to create a new identity, and looking forward to the future and setting new goals. It is well accepted in clinical practice and research that aphasia affects a person's sense of self. The self is defined by experiences of the past and present, and with expectations for the future, is dependent on social interaction and requires memory abilities (Brumfitt, 1993). Through regular involvement in core roles (teacher, dancer, etc.), the self develops a sense of identity in relation to other people (Brumfitt, 1993). For people with aphasia, the loss of speech, which is core to humanity, and the loss of language to talk through the change (Brumfitt, 1993), is the double impact of aphasia on sense of self.

Finally, self-esteem is frequently associated with PWB, and is 'an individual's judgement of overall self-worth, self-regard or self-acceptance' (Vickery, 2006, p. 1075). Self-esteem is thus one of the six dimensions in Ryff's PWB concept. A specific tool to measure this is the Visual Analogue Self-Esteem Scale (VASES: Brumfitt and Sheeran, 1999; see Chapter 4 of this text), which is gaining popularity with increasing use in small-scale evaluation studies in England (Ross, Winslow, Marchant and Brumfitt,

2006) and large-scale correlational and descriptive studies in the USA (see Vickery, 2006, for an inpatient rehabilitation study).

To summarise, there are many variables associated with well-being, which suggests that in any evaluation of a client's well-being the professional would be wise also to consider measuring the variables. There is evidence to suggest that the variables themselves correlate and influence each other, and no clear pattern of causation can be made. Thus, professionals need to be aware of the associations between emotional state and PWB; depression and limited socialisation; social activities and well-being; mood and goal achievement; as well as autonomy, competence, meaning and significance of clients' activities; and finally, identity; self-esteem and goal setting in their own right.

## Measuring well-being

This section of the chapter will explore the main drivers for measuring the well-being of adults with communication impairments, and discuss issues that need to be considered in measurement. A number of different measures are presented, and their potential to evaluate and explore clients' well-being is reviewed. To conclude the chapter, some specific recommendations are made for measuring well-being in adults with acquired communication impairments.

### Measuring the well-being of people with acquired communication impairments

> If changes in subjective well-being are to be considered in their own right as a result of conditions that lead to disablement, then the empirical relationships of subjective well-being to impairment, disability, and handicap, need to be established
>
> *(Fuhrer, 1996, p. 56)*

Clinicians and researchers have assumed that people's well-being is altered with the onset of stroke and communication disability, yet little empirical research has been conducted to indicate which consequences are most important, and thus most predictive of later functioning. Fuhrer conducted a review of 19 studies of people with spinal cord injury and found that SWB was commonly associated (correlated and predicted) with measures of handicap, inconsistently associated with disability, and minimally associated with impairments (Fuhrer, 1996). Speech and language therapists infrequently assess at the level of handicap or participation in rehabilitation, as measures are not communication-specific at this level. Fuhrer's finding should provoke discussion about how professionals consider the well-being of patients or clients who have multiple impairments, such as hemiplegia and dysarthria/aphasia. There is, however, very little multidisciplinary research conducted in adult acquired conditions, which would inform the investigation of whether the effects of multiple impairments and disabilities on well-being are additive, or whether there is synergy involved. Most professionals are typically concerned with measuring the impact of their discipline's involvement on the patient or client's well-being, which is based on the assumption that changes in well-being are attributed to changes in 'body structures and functions' (impairments) and 'activities'. Given the limited evidence base in this area, there is great scope for future research to explore the relative contribution of differing impairments and disabilities to well-being.

In aphasiology, research has already attempted to produce an empirical operational model for communication-related QoL in older adults with chronic aphasia (Cruice, Worrall, Hickson and Murison, 2003). Using 13 different measures assessing communication functioning, activity and participation, emotional health, PWB and HRQoL, the research illustrated that communication is not a determinant of health and that a sole generic HRQoL focus is inappropriate for people with aphasia (Cruice, Worrall, Hickson and Murison, 2003). QoL for older adults with chronic aphasia was more appropriately conceptualised as PWB as well as social HRQoL. Both of these variables were strongly predicted by the individuals' language and functional communication abilities.

Both UK professional bodies concerned with stroke and speech and language therapy emphasise the importance of well-being in rehabilitation. According to the Royal College of Physicians' second edition of guidelines for stroke (Royal College of Physicians, 2004, p. 26), the aims of rehabilitation are:

1. to maximise the patient's social rehabilitation;
2. to maximise the patient's sense of well-being (QoL) (and maximise satisfaction with life);
3. minimise stress on and distress of the family.

Other definitions within rehabilitation focus jointly on improving QoL through maximising the individual's functioning and attaining the highest level of well-being. For most clinicians, the real interest in measuring well-being is to gain the client's perspective in rehabilitation and ensure that interventions are as relevant to the client's needs, goals and desires as possible. This relationship between well-being and the needs, goals and desires of rehabilitation often remains unarticulated, and needs to be addressed more in both practice and research.

The Royal College of Speech and Language Therapists' (RCSLT) clinical guidelines for aphasia also reiterate the importance of well-being, stating that the aim of rehabilitation is 'to maximise the individual's sense of well-being/quality of life and their social position/roles' (Royal College of Speech and Language Therapists, 2005, p. 98). Review of the clinical guidelines for dysarthria suggests clinicians are to evaluate the emotional, psychological and psychosocial impact of the dysarthria for both the individual and the family (p. 95). In order to promote PWB, the RCSLT recommends 'an assessment and monitoring of changes in lifestyle; experience of loss and adjustment; the effect on relationships; changes in behaviour; emotional responses; attitudes; perceptions and socialisation . . . using a variety of tools and quality-of-life measures' (Royal College of Speech and Language Therapists, 2005, p. 95). Recent work by Walshe (2002, 2004) in the UK confirms the importance of the psychosocial impact and self-concept of adults with dysarthria (by stroke as well as other neurological issues).

Within the UK there is a strong sense amongst practitioners and researchers that psychosocial aspects are crucial to management and outcomes in intervention in aphasia (Brumfitt, 2006), suggesting that practice does indeed reflect the clinical guidelines within the speech and language therapy profession. However, actual well-being assessments are infrequently used. Only 39% of the respondents (total sample of 173) used published scales or methods to obtain information about psychosocial aspects in aphasia, and these included measures of depression and anxiety, self-esteem, QoL, communication disability and optimism, as well as visual elicitation methods. Alternatively, there was a strong preference for informal scales, used by 98% of respondents, and communicative history form, used by 80% of the respondents. Respondents raised the lack of clinical resources and lack of standardised measures as barriers to providing intervention for psychosocial aspects (Brumfitt, 2006).

In North America, the findings of actual practice are less encouraging. Simmons-Mackie, Threats and Kagan (2005) conducted an online survey of outcome assessment in aphasia with 94 respondents completing the survey in America (five from Canada). Only 14 of the 336 (4.2%) assessment tools or methods mentioned by respondents (interviews, observation, and conversation analyses included) related in any way to well-being or HRQoL. There were seven references to satisfaction surveys, four to QoL assessments, and three to affect and mood scales. This contrasts with 79 references to functional communication assessments (23.5%) and 153 references to linguistic and/or cognitive assessments (45.5%). It is possible that many clinicians recognise that the significant difficulties in measuring well-being with communication-impaired clients, and are waiting for more accessible tools to be developed. It is also possible that clinicians in fact *do use* well-being or QoL instruments in their practice, but use them as information-gathering tools rather than outcome measures, and hence did not report them in the survey. In the following section, the key issues that pertain to evaluation or measurement are considered.

## Measurement issues for consideration

The concerns in HRQoL measurement, as identified by Ebrahim (1995), are equally valid in measurement of well-being. Ebrahim identified that *repeatability* is problematic as the measure is often imprecise. This can be caused by variability, which is inherent in the measure, or caused by the problems in attributing changes—i.e. because of treatment and progression of disease, the individual's situation is likely to change. The *content validity*, specifically relevance to patients or clients, is problematic, with many measures being borrowed from other fields and not tested with clinical populations to explore their ability to capture what is meaningful to clients. The *sensitivity* of the measure is important, and includes its ability to discriminate and detect change in severity of the disease state, and sensitivity to rehabilitation services. Finally, *criterion validity*, which refers to whether the questionnaire measures what it intends to measure, can be problematic. It is important to note as well that 'tests are not inherently valid—they are valid only for a purpose, a range and a sample' (Tate, Dijkers and Johnson-Greene, 1996, p. 5).

Clearly, more research needs to be undertaken with adults with acquired communication impairments, their family members and friends, and service providers, to address the content and sensitivity of well-being measures. Until that evidence is created though, there are several key issues that professionals can consider when choosing from existing measures. It is recommended that speech and language therapists (SLTs) and clinical psychologists work together in considering appropriate measurement tools, each contributing their appropriate expertise—clinical psychologists for in-depth knowledge of the tools, and SLTs for in-depth knowledge of the client's linguistic and communication abilities (Brumfitt and Barton, 2006). The areas for consideration are discussed in turn below:

- *Communication skills required for self-evaluation*: people with aphasic communication impairments are likely to have the most difficulty of all adult communication-impaired persons in participating in well-being assessment. Complex linguistic skills are required of people to understand the questions, reflect on their meaning and then their lives, and finally express thoughts or choose from given options, and those skills will be impaired through aphasia. Speech and language therapists are well placed to advise on the likely linguistic complexity of well-being measures, and may have already identified questions or wording that are problematic from previously administering measures with clients. Preliminary small-scale studies indicate that some tools are more accessible for aphasic respondents than others (Cruice, Hirsch, Worrall, Holland and Hickson, 2000; Brady, 2007; Henson, 2007), but firm evidence is lacking and more research is urgently needed.
- *Index or aggregate measure (single score) versus profile measure*: the former may be more useful and concise for reporting well-being; however,

it can obscure meaningful data when results are collapsed into a single score; the latter provides a more complete picture of the individual, and can also enable change in one area to be more easily identified.

- *Single versus battery approach*: the former is cost effective, time efficient, easier to administer and score, whereas the latter is typically one measure for each dimension of interest and as such is the antithesis of the benefits listed above. Few complete measures of subjective well-being exist, thus a battery of satisfaction and affect measures are more likely. If using a battery approach, professionals need to be cautious when comparing measures because they frequently have different time referents (e.g. in the last week, compared to last month, etc.). Furthermore, some questions ask about the presence or absence of X whereas others ask about the impact of X on functioning, and there can be problems in scoring because of aggregation and unequal intervals (Barofsky in Spilker, 1996).

- *Content of the measure*: many measures evaluate the negative impact only, or are biased in some way for reporting more negative than positive aspects of well-being. For example, the Visual Analog Mood Scales (VAMS: Stern, 1997) has two positive mood scales (energetic, happy) and six negative mood scales (afraid, confused, sad, angry, tired, and tense). Professionals are encouraged to evaluate more than depression, distress and anxiety.

- *Responsiveness of the measure*: relatively few measures have been well tested to determine their responsiveness, i.e. their capacity to detect change. There is no literature available on responsiveness in well-being, therefore HRQoL is referred to. Generally speaking, a change of 0.5 on a 7-point Likert scale on a HRQoL measure is considered a minimal clinically significant difference (MCSD) or minimal clinically important difference (MCID) (see Jaeschke, Singer and Guyatt, 1989; Juniper, Guyatt, Willam and Griffith, 1994). With a 0–100 scale, this 0.5 difference translates to approximately 8 points (Sloan, Symonds, Vargas-Chanes and Fridley, 2003). It is important to note too that it can be hard to interpret change when we have no firm understanding of what a gold standard criterion should be in well-being. Note, the author is not suggesting there should be a gold standard though.

- *Response shift*: as Muldoon, Barger, Flory and Manuck (1998) state, 'the internal standard by which patients appraise their current state *shifts* and the same questionnaire items on well-being can elicit fundamentally different answers over time' (p. 544). Shifts in internal standards can occur purely as a function of time, as a function of onset of illness and/or disability, and also in relation to a change in level of functioning. Measures do not typically elicit how and why a person makes a decision about their well-being, and as such, this valuable information goes undocumented. Readers wanting further information on response shift are directed to the paper by Allison, Locker and Feine (1997) on quality of life as a dynamic construct.

- *Response options*: the purpose of measurement, be it predictive (adequate to predict criterion standard), evaluative (sufficient gradations are needed to register within-patient change) or discriminative (adequate response options to achieve fine or coarse discrimination depending on goals), affects the response options in measures (Juniper *et al.*, in Spilker, 1996). Measures that use agreement scales (strongly disagree–strongly agree) are problematic for aphasic respondents and yes/no judgements appear more reliable (Cruice, Hirsch, Worrall, Holland and Hickson, 2000), particularly for those respondents with poorer comprehension ability (Wernicke's or Conduction type aphasic profiles).
- *Dynamic nature of well-being*: one of the greatest problems is the dynamic nature of the well-being. Everything is in a constant flux, i.e. the person changes, the environment changes, and the interaction between the person and environment changes. Furthermore, perceptions and satisfaction often change as aims of treatment. This has been poorly appreciated in research and practice.

Finally, measuring well-being calls for special consideration of how comparisons are being made in the mind of the individual. Three types of comparisons can be made (Evans, 1994): firstly, a comparison between the current situation and the expected situation; secondly, a comparison of actual functioning (or achievements) relative to the individual's aspirations or potential; and thirdly, a comparison between achieved goals and unmet needs. Very rarely are these things considered in well-being measurement, and nor are researchers clear about the comparisons they ask participants to make when completing measures. For people with acquired communication impairments after stroke, there are three further bases for comparison: current state with premorbid state; current state with initial post-stroke state; and current state compared to peers with acquired communication impairments after stroke. People with aphasia who use the second or third comparisons are more likely to have higher quality of life than those who use the first (Cruice, 2001).

## A review of measurement instruments

> Are the life areas and changes in those life areas that are important to adults with acquired communication impairments and their families captured by instruments that we currently use in research and clinical practice?

This is a challenging question, and one that we do not yet know the answer to. The knowledge base is only beginning to develop, and qualitative research with respondents with communication impairments is only beginning to be more widely acceptable. We can, however, start with what we do know from the generic field of well-being outcome measurement, and predict what instruments may be useful for professionals working with adults with acquired communication impairments. Measures of well-being will be discussed first, followed by measures of emotional health.

Measures of well-being can be based on cognitive judgement or use the emotional-affective process as the foundation for evaluation. A combination of the cognitive and affective processes will yield a complete picture of subjective well-being. Readers wanting more information about each measure's psychometrics and an illustration of each tool are directed to the text *Measuring Health: A Guide to Rating Scales and Questionnaires* (McDowell and Newell, 1996). Readers wanting comprehensive information on the relevance of depression measures after stroke are referred to Bennett and Lincoln's 2004 report for the Stroke Association of the UK, entitled 'Screening for depression after stroke'. An abbreviated version of this appears as Bennett and Lincoln (2006).

Measures based on cognitive judgements include the Four Single Item Indicators of Well-being scale (see McDowell and Newell, 1996), Quality of life index (Ferrans and Powers, 1985), Satisfaction with life scale (Diener, Emmons, Larsen and Griffin, 1985), and the Life Satisfaction Index (Neugarten, Havighurst and Tobin, 1961). These measures are considered generic tools, and thus not specific to the consequences of the impact of acquired communication impairments on people's lives. The general consensus in the well-being and HRQoL field is a generic measure supplemented with a disease-specific measure. The Life Satisfaction Index A (see Neugarten, Havighurst and Tobin, 1961) has been frequently used with spinal cord populations, and is a 20-question assessment intended to tap distinct dimensions of life satisfaction, zest and apathy, resolution and fortitude, and congruence between desired and achieved goals (Fuhrer, 1994). It gives a single total score. It is important to note that satisfaction is comparative, depends on expectations, and is influenced by context.

Measures using the emotional-affective process as foundation include the Beck Depression Inventory (BDI: Beck, Ward, Mendelssohn and Erbaugh, 1961), the Rosenberg Self Esteem scale (RSE: Rosenberg, 1979), and the Profile of Mood States (POMS: McNair, Lorr and Droppleman, 1971) (see also Tate, Dijkers and Johnson-Greene, 1996). In short, the BDI takes both a cognitive and affective approach to measuring depression, but is reportedly not good at indicating clinical depression. Nor is it recommended for routine clinical practice with communication-impaired patients as its items are lengthy and complex, the response options change between items, and there are no cut-offs provided for stroke (Bennett and Lincoln, 2006). The POMS seems to fare much better and measures six moods, yielding a score of distress. It does, however, require the respondent to read through 60+ adjectives that represent the mood dimensions (depression/dejection; tension/anxiety; anger/hostility; vigour/activity;

fatigue/inertia; and confusion/bewilderment). This suggests a high level of respondent burden for communication-impaired respondents. The RSE is brief, unidimensional, and global, and measures self-worth and self-acceptance. Some people consider self-esteem as a substitute for life satisfaction (Tate, Dijkers and Johnson-Greene, 1996), yet others maintain it is an affective component (George and Bearon, 1980; Tate, Dijkers and Johnson-Greene, 1996). A review of multiple measures of depression and anxiety after stroke proposed that the Stroke Aphasic Depression Questionnaire-H10 (Lincoln, Sutcliffe and Unsworth, 2000) is the most appropriate measure for measuring depression in stroke patients with and without communication problems in hospital (Bennett and Lincoln, 2006). It comprises 10 items that are scored based on behaviours associated with mood that are observed by a carer. The timeframe reflects its relevance to the hospital situation: 'every day this week' to 'not at all this week'.

One widely used measure of PWB in social surveys and clinical populations in speech and language therapy is the Affect Balance Scale (ABS: Bradburn, 1969) of mental health, which independently taps quality, quantity and positive to negative balance of affect, in the past week (George, 1981). The ABS has been used to measure the effect of a communication partners' programme for 10 adults with aphasia, but was reported to show no significant change on post-treatment testing (Lyon et al., 1997). It is not uncommon, however, for group data to obscure real changes for specific individuals in the treatment study. Hemsley and Code (1996) also noted *individual* patterns of emotional and psychosocial adjustment for five aphasic participants who had similar types and severity of aphasia. Furthermore, Ross, Winslow, Marchant and Brumfitt (2006) noted individual but not group change on two measures of psychological well-being in seven aphasic participants. Other research suggests that the ABS is useful in measurement outcomes from group therapy with members with aphasia (Elman and Bernstein-Ellis in Holland and Thompson, 1998).

The General Health Questionnaire-28 (Goldberg, 1979) has been used to measure [subjective] well-being in stroke (Sveen et al., 2004) and aphasia (Hilari, Byng and Pring, 2001), yet the measure is described as a screening for short-term minor psychiatric disorder. Other researchers refer to the GHQ as a measure of psychological morbidity, mental health and psychological well-being. The 12-item version of the GHQ is specifically recommended as a short screening measure for depression after stroke, but as in nearly every single tool described here, requires further research with stroke patients (Bennett and Lincoln, 2006).

Steiner and colleagues (1996) discuss the Short Sense of Coherence Scale (see Antonovsky, 1993) with its 13 items, which is touted as a measure of psychological well-being. This scale purports to measure a stable psychological orientation that is hypothesised to be associated with both vitality and the capacity to identify and draw upon internal and external resources in the face of stressful situations. This measure has alternating positive and negative anchors, which can sometimes result in problems in completing the measure, and is likely to cause problems for language-impaired respondents. Steiner and colleagues also discuss the 15-item version of the Geriatric Depression Scale, which is a well-established measure for screening clinical depression in the elderly.

Possibly one of the greatest measures known is Carol Ryff's Psychological Well-being scale (Ryff, 1989), encompassing six dimensions of psychological well-being as self-acceptance, positive relations with others, autonomy, environmental mastery, purpose in life, and personal growth. Two subscales are perceived to relate to independence (autonomy and environmental mastery) and the remaining four relate to fulfilment. A short form of this scale contains 14 items per subscale (dimension), and a condensed version of the short form containing just four items per subscale was developed for the programme evaluation conducted in the York-Durham Aphasia Centre in the early 1990s (see Hoen, Thelander and Worsley, 1997). This preliminary study demonstrated that 35 people with aphasia and 12 relatives improved their psychological well-being over 6 months of attending the centre's programmes. It is also this shortened condensed version that demonstrated the importance of psychological well-being for participants with aphasia (Cruice, Worrall, Hickson and Murison, 2003).

The Communication Difficulty (CD), Communication-Associated Psychological Distress (CAPD), BOSS Negative Mood and BOSS Positive Mood scales hold significant potential for future studies exploring psychological aspects with aphasic clients (Doyle, McNeil, Hula and Mikolic, 2003). The CD scale is the longest with seven items: talk, understand what people say to you, understand what you read, write a letter, talk with a group of people, be understood by others, and find the words you want to say (Doyle, McNeil, Hula and Mikolic, 2003). The CAPD is comparatively short with three items only: how often do difficulties communicating (1) cause you to feel anxious, unhappy or frustrated; (2) cause you to feel dissatisfied with yourself or your life; and (3) prevent you from doing the things in life that are important to you? The mood scales are well balanced, with four negative items (lonely, anxious, angry and sad) and four positive items (confident, happy, calm and optimistic about the future).

The Visual Analog Mood Scales (VAMS: Stern, 1997) were developed specifically for post-stroke aphasic patients, to address the barriers of other measures: length, and linguistic, cognitive, memory and attention demands (Stern, 1999), and are described in detail in Chapter 6 of this text. Whilst the VAMS has vertical scale orientation accommodating possible hemianopia or neglect disturbances, which can influence the patient's self-report, it is the author's experience that respondents with chronic aphasia struggle to identify their QoL states on vertical lines.

Finally, the Rivermead Life Goals Questionnaire (Wade, 1999) can be used with stroke patients to determine the importance of nine key life areas to the individual patient. These life areas include: residential and domestic arrangements; personal care; leisure; work; relationship with partner; family life; contacts with friends, neighbours and acquaintances; religion/life philosophy; and financial status. Whilst there is much clinical support for this measure, this author stresses that the questionnaire does not exactly assess life goals, but rather the importance of life areas to the person. The language is not couched in goal wording, and there is no specific level to achieve, for example, 'my leisure, hobbies and interests including pets are: of no importance, of some importance, of great importance, of extreme importance'. The tool is useful, however, in ascertaining patient or client perspectives in terms of importance.

## Measurement recommendations

It seems clear from research and practice that no single measure will suit all circumstances and purposes for well-being evaluation. Therefore, it is impossible to recommend any one measure. Instead, a number of principles are recommended for measuring well-being with adults with acquired communication impairments:

- Choose measures that tap both positive and negative aspects of an individual's well-being.
- Where possible, choose measures that enable the patient's satisfaction *and/or* importance of each domain to be documented. If this is not possible, clinicians and researchers are encouraged to extend the evaluation with the person and discuss how satisfied she/he is and determine what is important.
- Multidimensional measures or a battery of unidimensional measures are recommended, because using a single outcome measure can lead professionals to make incorrect conclusions about the impact of a condition or treatment on someone's well-being (Birren, Lubben, Cichowlas Rowe and Deutchman, 1991). Multidimensional measures also provide more complete pictures (Fletcher, Dickinson and Philp, 1992).
- Likert scales, particularly the seven-point scale, are deemed easier to administer and easier to interpret than a visual analogue scale with undefined points (Juniper *et al.*, in Spilker, 1996).
- Measures must be completed using a face-to-face interviewer-assisted format, spoken aloud with the written measure available to read through simultaneously.
- Measures are best administered by a speech and language therapist who is trained on the measure and knowledgeable in techniques for maximising clients' understanding and expression (Cruice *et al.*, 2000).

The following features are considered desirable in well-being evaluation with people with aphasia (Cruice, 2001), but would need to be verified in further study:

- measures of approximately 10 minutes duration for administration;
- simple, clear and brief instructions;
- simple and/or consistent questions;
- consistent format of responses, preferably yes/no;
- horizontal rating scales, if they are used at all;
- response scales with defined points (not visual analogue); and
- clear layout, specifically, one question per page of assessment, with response scale repeated on each page; both printed in 18-point Times New Roman font.

In addition to the above, Hirsch and Holland (2000) suggest two further strategies: (1) careful ordering of items (e.g. all communication items together); and (2) instructions on each page, to reduce the demands on the person's memory.

## The 'gap principle'

This chapter has focused on the construct of well-being and the measurement of it, and yet has thus far ignored the important clinical question of how do we improve someone's well-being, i.e. what is the mechanism for changing and increasing a patient or client's well-being? As a last word before concluding this chapter, it seems appropriate to raise this issue, and suggest that it may be met by considering what is known as the 'gap principle' (Calman, 1987; Parmenter, 1994). The gap principle refers to the gap between someone's achievements and his or her expectations. It has also been used to describe the gap or comparison between someone's achievements and a third party's evaluation of that person's achievements. Taking the former example, the larger the gap between a person's achievements and their expectations, the lower their personal satisfaction and well-being is likely to be. Conversely, the smaller the gap between achievements and expectations, the greater their satisfaction and subsequently their well-being will be. It follows then that the aim of rehabilitation or any intervention is to narrow the gap. This is most likely undertaken by working on either or both of the person's *achievements* by providing speech and language therapy services targeting language, communication, participation, and by working on their *expectations*, such as counselling within speech and language therapy remit for adjustment and acceptance (when clinicians have had further training) or referral for specialist counselling services from clinical psychology.

## Conclusions

Improving quality of life is the primary motivation for speech and language therapists and other professionals intervening in the lives of adults with acquired communication impairments. Whilst physical health and social health are undeniably important in quality of life, it is well-being—achieving a sense of life satisfaction and happiness—that resonates more with the feelings and subsequent experiences of adults who have acquired some form of communication impairment.

It seems that regardless of whether the impairment is in language or speech, the impact on adults' social, emotional and psychological lives and their self-identity is similar. Maximising well-being in quality of life is forward looking, and focuses the person and the professional on narrowing the gap between the person's current achievements and desired aspirations, achieving happiness whilst reducing anxiety, depression and distress, and cultivating a positive mental attitude. New questionnaires and scales are being developed and validated as the role of well-being in quality of life increases in prominence, and will enable clinicians and researchers better to address adults' well-being in rehabilitation and community interventions. Clinicians and researchers across disciplines are encouraged to collaborate in the ongoing endeavour to make tools more accessible and relevant for people with acquired communication impairments, enabling people to have their say in their own evaluation.

## References

Allison P, Locker D, Fein J. Quality of life: a dynamic construct. Soc Sci Med 1997;45: 221–230.

Antonovsky A. The structure and properties of the Sense of Coherence scale. Soc Sci Med 1993;36:725–733.

Baldwin S, Godfrey C, Propper CE. Quality of Life: Perspectives and Policies. London: Routledge, 1990.

Baylor C, Yorkston K, Eadie T. The consequences of spasmodic dysphonia on communication-related quality of life: A qualitative study of the insider's experiences. J Commun Disord 2005;38:395–419.

Bays C. Quality of life of stroke survivors: A research synthesis. J Neurosci Nurs 2001;33: 310–316.

Bearon LB. Editorial: Conceptualizing quality of life: Finding the common ground. J Appl Gerontol 1988;7:275–278.

Beck AT, Ward CH, Mendelssohn MJ, Erbaugh J. An inventory for measuring depression. Arch Gen Psychiatr 1961;4:561–571.

Bennett H, Lincoln N. Screening for depression and anxiety after stroke: A review of potential measures for routine screening. Int J Therap Rehabil 2006;13:401–406.

Birren JE, Lubben JE, Cichowlas Rowe J, Deutchman DE. The Concept and Measurement of Quality of Life in the Frail Elderly. San Diego, CA: Academic Press, 1991.

Bradburn N. The structure of Psychological Well-being. Chicago, IL: Aldine, 1969.

Brady S. Self-reporting on Quality of Life: Measuring Limiting Factors in Clinical Assessments for People with Aphasia. Unpublished MSc dissertation. London: Department of Language and Communication Science, City University, 2007.

Brumfitt S. Losing your sense of self: What aphasia can do. Aphasiology 1993;7:569–575.

Brumfitt S. Psychosocial aspects of aphasia: Speech and language therapists' views on professional practice. Disabil Rehabil 2006;28:523–534.

Brumfitt S, Barton J. Evaluating wellbeing in people with aphasia using speech therapy and clinical psychology. Int J Therap Rehabil 2006;13:305–310.

Brumfitt S, Sheeran P. The development and validation of the visual analogue self-esteem scale (VASES). Brit J Clin Psychol 1999;38:387–400.

Calman K. Definitions and dimensions of quality of life. In:. Aaronson NK, Beckmann J (eds) The Quality of Life of Cancer Patients. New York: Raven, 1987; pp. 1–9.

Cruice M. Communication and Quality of Life in Older People with Aphasia and Healthy Older People. Unpublished PhD dissertation. Brisbane: Department of Speech Pathology and Audiology, University of Queensland, 2001.

Cruice M, Hill R, Worrall L, Hickson L. Conceptualising quality of life for older people with aphasia. Aphasiology (in press).

Cruice M, Hirsch F, Worrall L, Holland A, Hickson L. Quality of life for people with aphasia: Performance on and usability of quality of life assessments. Asia Pac J Speech Lang Hearing 2000;5:85–91.

Cruice M, Worrall L, Hickson L, Murison R. Finding a focus for quality of life with aphasia: Social and emotional health, and psychological well-being. Aphasiology 2003;17:333–353.

Cruice M, Worrall L, Hickson L. Perspectives of quality of life by people with aphasia and their family: Suggestions for successful living. Top Stroke Rehab 2006;13:14–24.

Cruice M, Worrall L, Hickson L. (2006b) Quantifying aphasic people's social lives in the context of their non-aphasic peers. Aphasiology;20(12):1210–1255.

Diener E, Emmons R, Larsen R, Griffin S. The satisfaction with life scale. J Pers Assess 1985;49: 71–75.

de Haan RJ, Limburg M, Van der Meulen JHP, Jacobs HM, Aaronson NK. Quality of life after stroke: Impact of stroke type and lesion location. Stroke 1995;26:402–408.

Doyle P, McNeil M, Hula W, Mikolic J. The Burden of Stroke Scale (BOSS): Validating patient-reported communication difficulty and associated psychological distress in stroke survivors. Aphasiology 2003;17:291–304.

Ebrahim S. Clinical and public health perspectives and applications of health-related quality of life measurement. Soc Sci Med 1995;41:1383–1394.

Engell B, Huber W, Hütter B. Quality of life measurement in aphasic patients. Proceedings of the 24th International Association of Logopaedics and Phoniatrics Congress, Amsterdam, August 1998.

Evans D. Enhancing quality of life in the population at large. Soc Indic Res 1994;33:47–88.

Fallowfield L. The Quality of Life: The Missing Measurement in Healthcare. London: Souvenir Press (E & A) Ltd, 1990.

Felce D, Perry J. Quality of life: Its definition and measurement. Res Dev Disabil 1995;16: 51–74.

Ferrans C, Powers M. Quality of life index: Development and psychometric properties. Adv Nurs 1985;8:15–24.

Fiori K, Antonucci T, Cortina K. Social network typologies and mental health among older adults. J Gerontol Psychol Sci Soc Sci 2006;61:25–32.

Fletcher A, Dickinson E, Philp I. Quality of life instruments for everyday use with elderly patients. Age Ageing 1992;21:142–150.

Fuhrer, M. Subjective well-being: Implications for medical rehabilitation outcomes and models of disablement. Am J Phys Med Rehab 1994;73:358–364.

Fuhrer M. The subjective well-being of people with spinal cord injury: Relationships to impairment, disability, and handicap. Top Spinal Cord Injury Rehab 1996;1:56–71.

George LK. Subjective well-being: Conceptual and methodological issues. In: Eisdorfer C (ed.) Annual Review of Gerontology and Geriatrics. New York: Springer, 1981; pp. 345–382.

George LK, Bearon LB. Quality of life in older persons: Meaning and measurement. New York: Human Sciences Press, 1980.

Goldberg D (1979). The General Health Questionnaire: GHQ-28. Psychological Medicine.

Hemsley G, Code C. Interactions between recovery in aphasia, emotional and psychosocial factors in subjects with aphasia, their significant others and speech pathologists. Disabil Rehabil 1996;18:567–584.

Henson A. Self-reporting on Quality of Life: Measuring Factors in Clinical Assessments for People with Aphasia. Unpublished MSc dissertation. London: Department of Language and Communication Science, City University, 2007.

Hilari K, Byng S. Measuring quality of life in people with aphasia: The Stroke Specific Quality of Life Scale. Int J Hum Commun Dis 2001;36(Suppl.):86–91.

Hilari K, Byng S, Pring T. Measuring well-being in aphasia: The GHQ-28 versus the NHP. Adv Speech-Lang Pathol 2001;3:129–137.

Hinckley J. Investigating the predictors of lifestyle satisfaction among younger adults with chronic aphasia. Aphasiology 1998;12:509–518.

Hinckley J. Finding messages in bottles: Living successfully with stroke and aphasia. Top Stroke Rehab 2006;13:25–36.

Hirsch F, Holland A. Beyond activity: Measuring participation in society and quality of life. In: Worrall L, Frattali C. (eds) Neurogenic Communication Disorders: A Functional Approach. New York: Thieme, 2000, pp. 35–54.

Hoen B, Thelander M, Worsley J. Improvement in psychological well-being of people with aphasia and their families: Evaluation of a community-based programme. Aphasiology 1997;11:681–691.

Holland A, Thompson C. Outcomes measurement in aphasia. In: Frattali C. (ed) Measuring Outcomes in Speech-Language Pathology. New York: Thieme, 1998.

Holland A, Frattali C, Fromm D. Communication Activities of Daily Living, 2nd edn. Texas: Pro-Ed, 1999.

Jaeschke R, Singer J, Guyatt GH. Measurement of health status. Ascertaining the minimal clinically important difference. Control Clin Trials 1989;10:407–15.

Juniper EF, Guyatt GH, Willam A, Griffith, LE. Determining a minimal important change in a disease-specific Quality of Life Questionnaire. J Clin Epidemiol 1994;47:81–87.

Kaplan RM, Anderson JP. The general health policy model: An integrated approach. In: Spilker B (ed.) Quality of Life in Pharmacoeconomics in Clinical Trials, 2nd edn. Philadelphia: Lippincott-Raven, 1996; pp. 309–322 (chapter 32).

Kertesz A. The Western Aphasia Battery. New York: Grune & Stratton, 1982.

Le Dorze G, Brassard C. A description of the consequences of aphasia on aphasic persons and their relatives and friends based on the WHO model of chronic diseases. Aphasiology 1995;9:239–255.

Lincoln NB, Sutcliffe LM, Unsworth G. Validation of the Stroke Aphasic Depression Questionnaire (SADQ) for use with patients in hospital. Neuropsychol Assess 2000;1:88–96.

Lundh U, Nolan M. Ageing and quality of life 1: Towards a better understanding. Brit J Nurs 1996;5:1248–1251.

Lyon J, Cariski D, Keisler L, Rosenbek J, Levine R, Kumpula J, Ryff C, Coyne S, Blanc M. Communication partners: Enhancing participation in life and communication for adults with aphasia in natural settings. Aphasiology 1997;11:693–708.

McDowell I, Newell C. Measuring Health: A Guide to Rating Scales and Questionnaires. 2nd edn. New York: Oxford University Press. 1996.

McKevitt C, Redfern J, La-Placa V, Wolfe C. Defining and using quality of life: A survey of healthcare professionals. Clin Rehabil 2003;17:865–870.

McNair D, Lorr M, Droppleman L. Manual for the Profile of Mood States. San Francisco: Education & Industrial Testing Service, 1971.

Menhert TH, Krauss KH, Nadler R, Boyd M. Correlates of life satisfaction in those with disabling conditions. Rehabil Psychol 1990;35:3–17.

Muldoon M, Barger S, Flory J, Manuck S. What are quality of life measurements measuring? BMJ 1998;316:542–545.

Nair K, Wade D. Life goals of people with disabilities due to neurological disorders. Clin Rehabil 2003;17:521–527.

Neugarten B, Havighurst R, Tobin S. The measurement of life satisfaction. J Gerontol 1961;16: 134–143.

Oishi S, Diener E, Suh E, Lucas R. Value as a moderator in subjective well-being. J Personality 1999;67:157–184.

Ozer M. Patient participation in the management of stroke rehabilitation. Top Stroke Rehab 1999;6:43–59.

Parmenter T. Quality of life as a concept and measurable entity. Soc Indic Res 1994;33: 9–46.

Pope AM, Tarlov AR. Disability in America: Towards a National Agenda for Prevention. Washington, DC: National Academy Press, 1991.

Records NL, Baldwin K. A tool to measure 'quality of life' of aphasic individuals. Paper presented at the 1996 ASHA Annual Convention, Pennsylvania.

Rosenberg M. Conceiving the Self. Malabar, FL: Robert E. Krieger, 1979.

Ross A, Winslow I, Marchant P, Brumfitt S. Evaluation of communication, life participation and psychological well-being in chronic aphasia: The influence of group intervention. Aphasiology 2006;20:427–448.

Ross K, Wertz R. Quality of life with and without aphasia. Aphasiology 2003;17:355–364.

Royal College of Physicians (RCP). National Clinical Guidelines for Stroke, 2nd edn. Prepared by the Intercollegiate Stroke Working Party. London: RCP, 2004.

Royal College of Speech and Language Therapists. RCSLT Clinical Guidelines. London: RCSLT, 2005.

Ryff C. Happiness is everything, or is it? Explorations on the meaning of well-being. J Pers Soc Psychol 1989;57:1069–1081.

Sarno M. Aphasia rehabilitation: Psychosocial and ethical considerations. Aphasiology 1993; 7:321–334.

Sarno M. Quality of life in aphasia in the first post-stroke year. Aphasiology 1997;11: 665–679.

Seed P, Lloyd G. Quality of Life. London: Jessica Kingsley, 1997.

Sheik J, Yesavage J. Geriatric Depression Scale (GDS): Recent evidence and development of a shorter version. Clin Gerontol 1986;5:165–172.

Simmons-Mackie N, Threats T, Kagan A. Outcome assessment in aphasia: A survey. J Commun Dis 2005;38:1–27.

Sloan J, Symonds T, Vargas-Chanes D, Fridley B. Practical guidelines for assessing the clinical significance of health-related quality of life changes within clinical trials. Drug Info J 2003;37:23–31.

Spilker B. (ed.) Quality of Life and Pharmacoeconomics in Clinical Trials, 2nd edn. Philadelphia: Lippincott-Raven, 1996.

Spilker B, Revicki D. Taxonomy of quality of life. In: Spilker B (ed.) Quality of Life and Pharmacoeconomics in Clinical Trials, 2nd edn. Philadelphia: Lippincott-Raven, 1996; pp. 25–32 (chapter 3).

Steiner A, Raube K, Stuck A, Aronow H, Draper D, Rubenstein L, Beck J. Measuring psychosocial aspects of well-being in older community residents: Performance of four short scales. The Gerontologist 1996;36:54–62.

Stern R. Visual Analog Mood Scales Manual. Psychological Assessment Resources, 1997.

Stern R. Assessment of mood states in aphasia. Semin Speech Lang 1999;20:33–50.

Sveen U, Thommessen B, Bautz-Holter E, Wyller T, Laake K. Well-being and instrumental activities of daily living after stroke. Clin Rehabil 2004;18:267–274.

Tate D, Dijkers M, Johnson-Greene L. Outcome measures in quality of life. Top Stroke Rehab 1996;2:1–17.

Tyerman A, Humphrey M. Changes in self-concept following severe head injury. Int J Rehabil Res 1984;7:11–23.

Van der Gaag A, Smith L, Davis S, Moss B, Cornelius V, Laing S, Mowles C. Therapy and support services for people with long-term stroke and aphasia and their relatives: A six-month follow-up study. Clin Rehabil 2005;19:372–380.

Vickery C. Assessment and correlates of self-esteem following stroke using a pictorial measure. Clin Rehabil 2006;20:1075–1084.

Wade D. Goal planning in stroke rehabilitation: How? Top Stroke Rehabil 1999;6:16–36.

Walshe M. 'You have no idea. You have no idea what it is like . . . not to be able to talk'. Exploring the Impact and Experience of Acquired Neurological Dysarthria from the Speaker's Perspective. Unpublished doctoral thesis. Dublin: Trinity College, 2002.

Walshe M. The impact of acquired neurological dysarthria on the speaker's self-concept. J Clin Speech Lang Stud 2004;12/13:9–33.

World Health Organization. WHOQOL Study Protocol (MNH/PSF/93.9). Geneva: WHO, 1993.

WHOQOL Group. Development of the World Health Organization WHOQOL-BREF Quality of Life Assessment. Psychol Med 1998;28:551–558.

Zemva N. Aphasic patients and their families: Wishes and limits. Aphasiology 1999;13: 219–234.

# 6 | The Visual Analog Mood Scales

## Robert A. Stern, Daniel Daneshvar, and Sabrina Poon

## Introduction

The assessment of psychological well-being in persons with neurological disorders in general, and with acquired communication impairments in particular, is a difficult and important task. This chapter provides an overview of the difficulties with differential diagnosis of mood disorders in these patient groups, followed by a discussion on the limitations of existing standardisd instruments that are used to evaluate mood changes and depression. As an appropriate alternative to other measurement techniques, the Visual Analog Mood Scales (VAMS; Stern, 1997) will be described, including their development, psychometric properties, previous relevant research, and recommendations for their use in clinical and research settings. Finally, new diagnostic categories for mood-related changes in patients with acquired communication disorders and other neurological conditions will be proposed.

### Disorders of mood associated with neurological illness

Neurological diseases and conditions are often accompanied by emotional and behavioural changes. The most prevalent of these neuropsychiatric conditions is depression and related mood disorders (Lyness, Niculescu, Tu, Reynolds and Caine, 2006). Symptoms of depression often present in patients with Alzheimer's disease (Starkstein and Mizrahi, 2006), stroke (Chemerinski and Levine, 2006), Huntington's disease (Hahn-Barma *et al.*, 1998), vascular disease (Barnes *et al.*, 2006), vascular dementia (Bowirrat, Oscar-Berman and Logroscino, 2006), Parkinson's disease (Rojo *et al.*, 2003), and traumatic brain injury (TBI) (Alderfer, Arciniegas and Silver, 2005). However, depression is widely underdiagnosed or misdiagnosed when it accompanies one of these neurological illnesses (Schubert, Burns, Paras and Sioson E, 1992; Bergdahl *et al.*, 2005; Gelenberg and Hopkins, 2007). This lack in diagnostic accuracy of mood disturbance in neurological conditions poses a significant public health problem, due to the association of depression with poorer health-related quality of life (Schrag, 2006), faster cognitive decline (Ganguli *et al.*, 2006; Steffens *et al.*, 2006), increased disability in activities of daily living and overall functional status (Lyness *et al.*, 1993; Alexopoulos *et al.*, 1996), increased social isolation

(Alexopoulos *et al.*, 2002), decreased rehabilitation outcome (Cully *et al.*, 2005), a higher rate of nursing home admission (Harris, 2007), greater use of nursing home resources (Smalbrugge *et al.*, 2006), and increased caregiver burden (Scazufca, Menezes and Almeida, 2002).

Post-stroke mood disorders are an important example of how far-reaching the public health impact may be. It has been estimated that between 20% and 40% of stroke patients develop some form of depression-like syndrome (Kotila, Numminen, Waltimo, and Kaste, 1998; Dam, 2001). In the USA, the prevalence of stroke in adults between 65 and 75 years of age is 6.2%, with the prevalence increasing to 12.5% for those 75 years and older (National Center for Health Statistics, 2005). Because of the tremendous growth internationally in the size of the elderly population in the coming decades, mood disturbance following stroke is likely to impact millions of individuals.

In order to provide appropriate and effective treatment for mood disorders associated with neurological illness, such as stroke, the mood disturbance must first be diagnosed accurately. However, depression is challenging to diagnose, especially when it accompanies a neurological disorder. First, depression following neurological illness may have multiple aetiologies. For example, Naarding and colleagues have suggested that, unlike patients with idiopathic depression, patients with depression due to vascular dementia may have three distinct presentations: patients with mood symptoms, those with psychomotor symptoms, and those with predominantly vegetative symptoms (Naarding *et al.*, 2003). Each of these subgroups may be directly related to a particular area or system of brain involvement and, as a result, each type may require specific treatment.

Another diagnostic issue related to the potential for neurological illnesses to mask or mimic depression is that depression often presents differently when it is comorbid with a neurological disorder. For instance, when patients with TBI have depression, they tend to display more aggression than patients who have not had TBI, thus complicating the diagnosis (Babin, 2003). Any valuable diagnostic tool must therefore take into account how depression presents differently in, and is sometimes masked or mimicked by, a neurological illness. The task of identifying patients with depression or other mood disorders in cases of neurological illness is made all the more complicated due to the lack of formal diagnostic criteria for psychiatric/neuropsychiatric conditions in patients with neurological disorders.

## Diagnosing depression in patients with acquired communication disorders

The diagnosis of Major Depressive Episode (MDE), according to *the Diagnostic and Statistical Manual of Mental Disorders, Fourth Edition, Text Revision* (*DSM-IV-TR*), will serve as a context from which the issues of diagnosing mood disorders in persons with aphasia will be explored. According to the *DSM-IV-TR*, to be diagnosed with MDE a patient must display symptoms of either depressed mood or loss of interest of pleasure (i.e. anhedonia). Additionally, a patient must have at least five of the following symptoms (American Psychiatric Association, 2000):

1. depressed mood most of the day;
2. markedly diminished interest or pleasure in almost all activities;
3. significant weight loss or weight gain;
4. insomnia or hypersomnia;
5. psychomotor agitation or retardation;
6. fatigue or loss of energy nearly every day;
7. feelings of worthlessness or inappropriate guilt;
8. diminished ability to think or concentrate, or indecisiveness;
9. recurrent thoughts of death or recurrent suicidal ideation.

**Neurobehavioural features associated with acquired communication disorders may mask or mimic the signs and symptoms of depression**

Both clinicians and caregivers often must evaluate a patient's outward expression of emotion, or affect, when determining a patient's internal mood state. In fact, clinicians often base their diagnoses primarily on these outward signs (Stern and Bachman, 1994). This approach is problematic in patients with neurological disorders in general, and even more so in patients with acquired communication impairments. The absence of direct verbal communication from a patient may lead a clinician to rely solely on outward expressions of emotion, which may not accurately reflect the patient's internal mood state. Discrepancies often exist between the assessment of the caregiver/clinician and the patient's self-report (Chemerinski *et al.*, 2001), and between the clinician's assessment and the caregiver's report (Kalpakjian, Lam and Leahy, 2002). This type of difficulty, as well as other similar impairments with differential diagnosis, will be presented below using the *DSM-IV* criteria for MDE.

1. *Depressed mood most of the day* Dysprosody, the impaired ability to produce fluctuations in melodic intonation in speech, often accompanies neurological disorders such as stroke (Carota, Staub and Bogousslavsky, 2002). These communication impairments are often mistaken by caregivers and clinicians for depressed mood (Rosenbek *et al.*, 2006). That is, the patient 'sounds depressed' due to flat or monotonic voice expression, even when his or her internal mood state might be quite different. The possibility of overlapping symptoms due to dysprosody must be carefully considered before a diagnosis of depression is made in any patient having suffered a stroke (Black, 1995).
Depressed mood may also be confused with the decreased facial expression that can be caused by neurological illnesses. For example,

patients with Alzheimer's disease often display diminished motor expression rates for speech and facial expressions (Scarmeas *et al.*, 2004). 'Masked facies', or extremely decreased facial expression, is a hallmark feature of Parkinson's disease (Simons, Pasqualini, Reddy and Wood, 2004). Because these patients are not externally displaying their internal mood state (i.e. their affect may be incongruent with mood), clinicians and caregivers may base their assessments on incomplete information.

2. *Markedly diminished interest or pleasure in almost all activities* Apathy, or the lack of emotional response or reactivity, can easily be confused with diminished interest or pleasure (Marin, 1990). Apathy is perhaps one of the most common neuropsychiatric features. For example, according to one study, apathy was observed in nearly 40% of patients with Alzheimer's disease, compared to none of the healthy controls (Starkstein, Petracca, Chemerinski and Kremer, 2001). Apathy, therefore, could be considered the neurological equivalent of the psychiatric anhedonia. However, in patients with neurological disorders, apathy can frequently exist in isolation from any other signs and symptoms of MDE. In addition to the direct effects that the neurological condition has on apathy, the indirect effects of an acquired neurological disorder can result in a diminished ability to perform previously enjoyable or pleasurable activities, due to either cognitive, motor or communication deficits. This change in behaviour must not be interpreted as a lack of interest, but rather a lack of ability.

3. *Significant weight loss or weight gain* Changes in eating behaviours and appetite can also accompany some neurological diseases, including Alzheimer's disease (Mirakhur *et al.*, 2004). These disturbances can lead to weight loss or gain, again mimicking a diagnostic criterion of MDE. Changes in weight may also be due directly to the neurological illness, or to either a concurrent medical illness or hospitalisation (Powell-Tuck and Hennessy, 2003).

4. *Insomnia or hypersomnia* There are several reasons for a patient with neurological disease to present with insomnia or hypersomnia besides depression. Common concurrent medical illnesses, such as diabetes, heart disease, sleep apnoea or hypothyroidism, or concurrent medications could lead to disruptions in the sleep–wake cycle in patients with neurological illnesses. Hospitalisation can also cause changes in sleep, effectively mimicking this symptom of MDE. One study that monitored sleep habits over a 3-month hospital stay found that chronic insomnia rates doubled from preadmission to discharge (Griffiths and Peerson, 2005). This increase in the prevalence of insomnia makes an accurate diagnosis of depression (based on this criterion) difficult in patients who are frequently hospitalised or who are still in their initial, acute hospitalisation or inpatient rehabilitation.

5. *Psychomotor agitation or retardation* The symptom of psychomotor retardation is shared by idiopathic depression and by neurological disorders. For example, a symptom most commonly associated with Parkinson's disease is bradykinesia, the slowing of movements due to the neurological condition. Bradykinesia can also be observed in patients with Alzheimer's disease and other neurodegenerative disorders (Kurz, 2005). One study indicated that the slowing of the thought process due to a neurological condition, or bradyphrenia, in Parkinson's disease and psychomotor retardation in depressive illness may also be closely related, as the dopaminergic pathway is impaired in both disorders (Rogers *et al.*, 1987). The terms 'psychomotor retardation' and 'bradyphrenia/bradykinesia' are, therefore, likely referring to the same or similar observed clinical presentations. However, the specific use of the terms is typically employed by psychiatrists and neurologists, respectively.

6. *Fatigue or loss of energy nearly every day* The issue of motivation complicates a clinician's or caregiver's perception of fatigue or loss of energy. Disorders affecting motivation occur frequently in individuals following TBI (Marin and Wilkosz, 2005) and other conditions. While the observer may assume that the patient wishes to continue characteristic behaviours but simply does not have the energy to do so, in many cases the patient's motivation may be influenced by neurological illness. Consequently, several neurological disorders present with symptoms that may be confused for fatigue or energy loss. For example, a patient with abulia, the neurological term for the loss of initiative or drive due to a neurological condition, may appear fatigued or at a loss of energy, as might be the case in idiopathic depression. However, the abulia, or perhaps, apathy, may merely make the individual appear to be fatigued outwardly (Marin, 1990).

7. *Feelings of worthlessness or inappropriate guilt* The criterion of worthlessness or guilt is dependent upon the ability of the patient accurately to communicate these thoughts to the clinician or caregiver. However, in patients with communication disorders, the observer may not be able to rely on verbal expression of these thoughts and, therefore, must be dependent upon the outward expression of emotion. As described above in greater detail, patients with a variety of neurological conditions may have impaired prosodic and facial expression of mood, thus resulting in a misinterpretation of their 'flat' affect as being overall dysphoric, which in turn could be extrapolated to having feelings of worthlessness and guilt.

In addition to diminished prosody and facial expression, many patients with neurological conditions present with extreme displays of affect, which further complicates the assessment of a patient's internal mood state. Some patients may exhibit mood-congruent emotional displays, such as TBI patients with orbitofrontal lesions and resulting disinhibition or exaggeration of the underlying emotional state (Arciniegas, Topkoff and Silver, 2000). This emotional disinhibition is also seen frequently in both Parkinson's disease and Alzheimer's disease (Mirakhur *et al.*, 2004; Lieberman, 2006). In fact, in one study of patients with Alzheimer's disease, 39% of patients showed pathological affect: 25% displayed crying episodes, and 14% showed laughing or mixed laughing and crying episodes (Starkstein *et al.*, 1995).

Other patients, such as those with pseudobulbar palsy, may exhibit the outward, motor expression of 'pathological' laughing or crying, but this outward expression is not representative or congruent with the underlying mood. An inaccurate interpretation of the patient's mood would understandably be made by the observer of the patient who appears to be crying, even though this motoric crying may be occurring in the presence of euthymic mood.

8. *Diminished ability to think or concentrate, or indecisiveness* Major depression is associated with changes in cognitive function. Although once believed to primarily be due to diminished effort, it is now widely accepted that the cognitive impairment in idiopathic MDE is, at least in part, secondary to the underlying neurochemical and neuropathological alterations in the disorder (Levin *et al.*, 2007). However, almost by definition, neurological conditions (e.g. dementia, TBI, stroke) have significant cognitive deficits as part of their overall presentation. Therefore, it is not possible to use this specific criterion as part of the differential diagnosis of MDE in patients with neurological disorders.

9. *Recurrent thoughts of death or recurrent suicidal ideation* Thoughts of self-harm, death, or suicidal ideation are a common and important indicator of MDE. However, patients with aphasia or other communication impairments that have difficulty expressing their feelings verbally may be especially prone to having their views misinterpreted. As stated above, without direct verbal communication, clinicians or caregivers are likely to base their assessment on external cues such as facial expression (Stern and Bachman, 1994).

As seen above, the diagnosis of MDE using traditional psychiatric criteria, such as the *DSM-IV*, is complicated and, perhaps, impossible in patients with neurological disorders in general, and in patients with aphasia and other communication disorders in particular. Mood disorders following an acquired neurological condition may often present quite differently than idiopathic mood disorders (Rigler, 1999). In addition, the signs and symptoms of the neurological condition may either mask or mimic the diagnostic criteria used for psychiatric mood disorders. Because of this difficulty, it would be helpful to establish new criteria for the diagnosis of mood disorders in neurological conditions that are based on the issues raised above, and on the specific neurobehavioural syndromes associated with neurological disorders. Box 6.1 presents this type of proposed nosology.

## Box 6.1 Proposed neuropsychiatric diagnostic classifications (modified from Stern, 1999)

- Apathetic/Abulic Disorder
- Emotional Disinhibition Disorder
- Agitation/Anxiety Syndrome
- Indifference/Undue Cheerfulness Syndrome
- Dysphoric Reaction
- Vegetative Depressive Syndrome
- Nondysphoric Depression
- Emotional Expression Disorder

## Standardised assessment of diagnosing depression in patients with acquired communication disorders

The difficulties in diagnosing depression based on clinician and caregiver observations in patients with neurological disorders warrant the need for standardised instruments either to measure overall syndromal depression or to determine a patient's internal mood state in this specific population. However, many of the available instruments are not tailored to patients with aphasia and related communication impairments, but are instead created for use with individuals with intact communication skills, cognitive capacity, memory, attention and affective display (Stern, 1996). Because these assumptions are not always valid in individuals with neurological impairments, some instruments have been modified or created for use specifically to evaluate mood state and depression in these patients. Still, many of these instruments have limitations due to the neurobehavioural impairments common in patients with an acquired communication disorder.

### Limitations due to non-fluent aphasia

Many instruments assess depression or mood by asking questions related to each of the nine possible symptoms of MDE. To avoid the difficulties of overlapping symptoms, some instruments designed for patients with neurological deficits make use of a structured interview, i.e. the Hamilton Depression Rating Scale (Hamilton, 1960), the Present State Examination (Lesage, Cyr and Toupin, 1991), and the Cornell Scale for Depression and Dementia (Alexopoulos, Abrams, Young and Shamoian, 1988). By utilising an interview, the clinician is able to determine whether specific symptoms are believed to be due to a neurological or physical illness, rather than a mood disorder.

While this structured interview may address many of the issues involved in diagnosing depression in patients with neurological disorders, there are additional complications in patients with communication impairments. Patients with non-fluent aphasia have difficulty providing meaningful responses to questions. Because interview-based assessments require the observer to rate mood items based on verbal output, these diagnostic questionnaires cannot be directly applied to individuals with non-fluent aphasia. As a result, such instruments are better suited for use on other patient populations, but are not useful for determining the mood state of patients with communication impairments.

### Limitations due to fluent aphasia

In order to avoid observer bias, some depression rating measures make use of a paper and pencil, or a yes or no response format, i.e. the Beck Depression Inventory (Schwab *et al.*, 1967), the Structured Assessment of Depression in Brain-Damaged Individuals (Gordon *et al.*, 1991), and the Zung Self-Rating Depression Scale (Wang, Treul and Alverno, 1975). By relying only on patient response for each item on the questionnaire, the validity of the instrument is preserved. However, these questionnaires require adequate reading and/or language skills. In patients with fluent aphasia, comprehension of spoken and written language is often compromised. Additionally, tasks such as adjective check lists require the ability to understand and choose among words or phrases. As a result, these written examinations are not well suited to determining depression in individuals with communication impairments.

### Limitations due to executive dysfunction

Stroke and other disorders may result in executive dysfunction (Cummings and Benson, 1988). The presence of executive dysfunction could affect a patient's ability accurately to respond to a standardised depression questionnaire. For example, a patient with significant executive dysfunction may have difficulty answering test items reliably, may exhibit a response bias due to perseveration, or may be unable to maintain the response set necessary to answer the question (Stern and Prohaska, 1996). Executive impairments are compounded by longer and more complicated scales, i.e. the Chicago Multiscale Depression Inventory (Nyenhuis *et al.*, 1998).

### Limitations due to memory impairment

Many of these oral and written scales make use of questions that ask how a patient has felt some time in the past. These questions help to obtain a more consistent impression of how the patient has felt over time. Many patients with acquired communication disorders, however, may also have acquired deficits in learning. For these patients, only questions regarding their current mood state or behaviours at the time of interview can be answered with any reliability.

### Limitations due to impaired emotional expression

Interview-based assessments have additional drawbacks when used for patients with communication impairments. As previously discussed, patients with neurological disorders may display dysprosodia, impaired facial expression or, perhaps, pathological displays of laughing and crying. Therefore, in a clinical interview, the clinician could be biased by either the lack of verbal emotional expression or the presence of extreme displays of affect.

In some cases, the written or yes/no depression scales are administered to a caregiver rather than the loved one, thus avoiding many of the issues resulting from the patient's non-fluent aphasia, executive dysfunction or memory impairment. However, these tests again rely on external indicators of emotional response, which are often incongruous with internal mood.

Depression diagnosis in patients with aphasia should always include a self-report of *subjective* symptoms of mood as it does in individuals without aphasia (Townend, Brady and McLaughlan, 2007). Moreover, recent research suggests that non-dysphoric depression (i.e. symptoms of MDE or dysthymia without sad mood or anhedonia) is common following right anterior stroke (Paradiso *et al.*, 2008), further supporting the need to obtain a measure of subjective mood state when assessing neuropsychiatric status in stroke patients.

## Visual analogue scales

To address the challenges outlined above, non-verbal mood scales have been developed to evaluate a patient's internal mood state. The typical visual analogue scale consists of a horizontal line, 100 mm in length, with opposite words, phrases or statements at each end of the line (Aitken, 1969; Folstein and Luria, 1973). The scale may have a question accompany each scale (i.e. 'How do you feel?') with opposite answers at each spectrum (i.e. 'Happy' or 'Sad'), or it may have a sentence at each end (i.e. 'I feel the worst I have ever felt,' 'I feel the best I have ever felt'). Although these scales are very different from one another with no standardised design or administration, they have been shown to be good indicators of mood state. Even when compared to multi-item scales, a single, global, quality of life visual analogue scale has been shown to have excellent validity and reliability (de Boer *et al.*, 2004). Because there are a number of visual analogue scales, an evaluation of several scales designed for patients with communication impairments is necessary.

### Visual Analog Dysphoria Scale

Visual analogue scales were first used to assess mood in post-stroke patients by Robinson and Benson (1981). A modification of this approach, the Visual Analog Dysphoria Scale (VADS), was developed by Stern and Bachman (1991). The VADS consists of a 100-mm vertical line with cartoon-like happy and sad faces on the top and bottom of the scale, respectively. The anchor words 'happy' and 'sad' are printed above or below the respective faces. Patients are instructed to indicate how they feel by placing a horizontal mark across the vertical line. Using a vertical scale avoids impairments of visual field defects or hemispatial neglect that sometimes follow stroke and other conditions. Instructions are either given by words, gestures or both words and gestures. The VADS is scored from 0 to 100 based on the distance from the top, 'happy' pole to the mark made by the patient.

The VADS has several advantages over other mood assessments. First, the VADS takes only seconds to complete and patients with impaired comprehension can usually understand the task and provide meaningful, valid results. The VADS is significantly correlated with other lengthier, cognitively challenging and linguistically demanding assessments (Stern and Bachman, 1991). Additionally, rather than a binary yes/no response, a graded response allows for the evaluation of smaller mood changes.

Although the results from the VADS were found to be valid measures of mood states in patients with communication impairments (Stern and Bachman, 1991) and have been used successfully in subsequent studies of post-stroke depression (e.g. Gainotti et al., 1997; Paolucci et al., 1999), there are several shortcomings. Because the VADS uses extreme emotions at either pole, a mark very close to one pole could represent either the presence of that emotion, or the absence of its opposite. For example, a score of 0 resulting from a mark at the top, 'happy' pole is not a clear indicator of mood state, as it could represent either extreme happiness, or the complete absence of sadness. Moreover, having only one scale limits the number of emotions than can be examined.

### The Depression Intensity Scale Circles

The Depression Intensity Scale Circles (DISCs) is another mood assessment tool for patients with neurological disorders, including brain injuries (Turner-Stokes, Kalmus, Hirani and Clegg, 2005). The DISCs uses a 15-cm vertical line with circles of 2 cm diameter centred at either pole. Along the line there are four additional circles, evenly spaced, of identical size. The six circles in total have an increasing proportion of dark shading from bottom to top. The tester, using either gestures, words, pictures or some combination of these methods, explains that the scale measures sadness or depression. Each grey circle indicates how sad or depressed the patient feels, with the bottom, clear circle showing no sadness or depression, and the top, fully shaded circle indicating the worst possible sadness or depression. The patient then indicates which circle best describes his or her internal mood state.

The DISCs shares many of the same advantages as the VADS. It is also a valid, reliable and responsive measure of depression that produces a graded response allowing tracking of smaller changes. By focusing on current emotions, it avoids concerns of memory impairment. Furthermore, by using shaded circles rather than words, it is more likely to be understood by a patient with language or communication difficulties.

While the DISCs is a promising indicator of mood, it too has limitations. First, because it utilises circles rather than faces, more explanation is required to convey the task; i.e. without the additional cartoon-like face depicting an emotion (as in the VADS), the scale cannot exploit the ability of individuals with aphasia to utilise their intact ability to comprehend the non-verbal cartoon. For a patient with executive dysfunction, this scale might also prove challenging in that the conceptualisation of the gradient must be accurate. Additionally, because it has two extremes and only one question (i.e. no sadness and worst sadness), the number of emotions being assessed is limited. Further discussion of DISCs can be found in Chapter 2.

### Visual Analog Mood Scales

### Description

Many of the limitations of other previously described instruments have been addressed in the Visual Analog Mood Scales (VAMS) (Stern 1996, 1997). The VAMS was created to provide an accurate diagnosis and assessment of internal mood state changes specifically for neurologically impaired patients, and especially for those with aphasia or other communicational deficits. The VAMS consists of eight scales with 100-mm vertical lines, each evaluating a different mood state (Box 6.2).

### Box 6.2    Visual Analog Mood Scales (VAMS): eight distinct measurements

- Sad
- Happy
- Tense
- Confused
- Afraid
- Energetic
- Tired
- Angry

Each scale displays a specific cartoon-like mood face at the bottom, and a neutral cartoon-like face at the top. The word 'neutral' is printed above the neutral face, and the name of the mood (i.e. 'sad', 'tense', etc.) is printed below the corresponding mood face. By printing the word along with the face, issues of impaired facial recognition are avoided. While the addition of a mood word also provides additional information for individuals who are able to interpret and retain the word, it is not necessary for completing the task. The patient places a horizontal mark across the line to indicate current mood state. This mark is converted to a 0–100 scale based on distance in millimetres from the top of the scale (i.e. neutral pole). Therefore, a score of 100 indicates extreme endorsement of the specific mood. The faces have a minimum number of features in order to avoid excessive subtleties and detail. Like the VADS, the VAMS also has a vertical orientation to accommodate patients who have neglect. Figures 6.1 and 6.2 depict the 'Sad' and 'Tense' scales respectively.

### Administration

Each VAMS scale is presented on its own page, allowing the scales to be presented individually or as a group. In this way, the examiner can investigate a specific research or clinical question, or obtain a generalised assessment of mood. The set of eight scales can be administered quickly, typically in under 4 minutes, even in patients with severe cognitive or linguistic deficits. The test booklet has printed instructions on the cover, so the test can be self-administered without an examiner. However, to avoid issues of reading comprehension, the exam can also be administered using the provided verbal and non-verbal instructions.

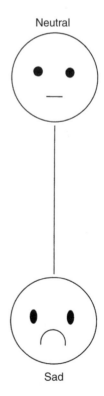

**Figure 6.1** The 'Sad' scale from the Visual Analog Mood Scales. Reproduced from Stern RA. Visual Analog Mood Scales. Lutz, FL: Psychological Assessment Resources, Inc., 1997, by special permission of the publisher.

Neutral

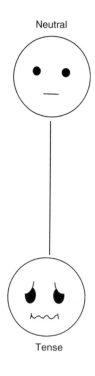

Tense

**Figure 6.2** The 'Tense' scale from the Visual Analog Mood Scales. Reproduced from Stern RA. Visual Analog Mood Scales. Lutz, FL: Psychological Assessment Resources, Inc., 1997, by special permission of the publisher.

In cases where respondents are unable to make an appropriate mark due to a motor difficulty (i.e. apraxia, hemiplegia or other motor disorders), alternative instructions are included. In these cases, the examiner would ask the patient to indicate which point best describes his or her current mood state while the examiner runs a finger along the line.

The examiner is also able to assess whether the respondent understands the tasks and is providing meaningful answers. While the vast majority of respondents are able to complete the task adequately, a respondent with severe executive dysfunction might not be capable of fulfilling the task. In these cases, alternative instructions included in the packet instruct the examiner to point at individual faces and ask binary questions (i.e. 'Are you sad?' when pointing at the sad face).

### Normative data

Normative data from over 400 healthy adult controls, 18–94 years old, is included with the VAMS test manual (Stern, 1997). The VAMS test manual also includes age- and gender-based T scores (i.e. standardised scores with a mean of 50 and SD of 10), as well as specific cut-off scores for screening of possible depression. The VAMS test manual also provides data from over 200 psychiatric inpatients and outpatients.

## Validation

Several validation studies have examined the VAMS with samples varied by age, neurological deficit (Nyenhuis *et al.*, 1997; Stern *et al.*, 1997; Turner-Stokes, Kalmus, Hirani and Clegg, 2005), psychiatric inpatients or outpatients (Stern, 1997), dementia patients (Temple *et al.*, 2004), and acute and post-acute stroke patients (Arruda, Stern and Somerville, 1999). These, and other studies, demonstrate the VAMS to have good convergent and discriminant validity (Arruda *et al.*, 1999). The VAMS has been shown to correlate with the Beck Depression Inventory (BDI), the Centre for Epidemiology Studies-Depression scale (CES-D), the Hamilton Depression Rating Scale (HDRS), and the Profile of Mood States (POMS), accounting for up to two-thirds of the variance of these lengthy, linguistically demanding and cognitively challenging tests. In a study of electroconvulsive therapy for the treatment of psychiatric depression, the VAMS was shown to have the same sensitivity to treatment effects as the lengthier, interview-based HDRS (Arruda, Stern and Legendre, 1996). The VAMS has also been recently used in several studies of elderly patients with dementia (e.g. Stern *et al.*, 2004; Bhalla, Papandonatos, Stern and Ott, 2007).

Case studies 6.1 and 6.2 are provided as examples of the use of the VAMS in clinical settings:

---

### Case Study 6.1 Reduced emotional expression mimicking depression

S.R. is a 76-year-old, right-handed widowed woman who had recently fallen and suffered bifrontal subdural haematomas. Following the evacuation of the haematomas she had residual dysarthria and mild word-finding impairments, as well as significantly reduced prosody and facial expression. She was discharged home to live with her adult daughter and her family. She had no prior history of depression. The daughter brought the patient to her weekly speech therapy appointment and told the therapist that she felt that her mother was 'severely depressed'. This concern was based on the patient's appearance of being 'down' and that, in contrast to her premorbid jovial style, she was now very 'flat' and did not seem to care about anything. The daughter was also concerned that her typically energetic mother slept much of the day. There was no report of weight loss and her night-time sleep schedule was similar to before the stroke. The speech and language therapist administered the VAMS to the patient, and her scores are given in Table 6.1.

**Table 6.1** VAMS scores for S.R.

|          | Afraid | Confused | Sad | Angry | Energetic | Tired | Happy | Tense |
|----------|--------|----------|-----|-------|-----------|-------|-------|-------|
| **Raw**     | 20     | 83       | 10  | 0     | 5         | 48    | 70    | 8     |
| **T-score** | 53     | 96       | 47  | 42    | 28        | 53    | 49    | 43    |

The VAMS indicated that S.R. felt significantly confused and reported a lack of energy (based on T-scores above or below one standard deviation [SD] of the normative group mean; i.e. T-scores >60 or <40). Self-reported sadness, fear, anger, tension, fatigue and happiness were all within normal limits based on the normative sample of women her age. Upon additional inquiry, the patient was able to acknowledge her sense of confusion since the fall and surgery, but was able to reassure her daughter that she was not 'depressed' or sad. With gains in speech and language treatment, she became more engaged in family activities. The daughter was also able to learn not to interpret her mother's lack of outward expression of emotion as the presence of sadness, but, rather, that it was due to the specific acquired brain damage and unrelated to mood state.

---

### Case Study 6.2 Expressive aphasia leading to difficulty in diagnosing depression

J.B. is an 82-year-old, right-handed married man who had a left middle cerebral artery stroke and a resulting profound non-fluent aphasia and dense right hemiparesis. He was transferred to a rehabilitation facility where he was receiving both speech and physical therapy. Prior to the stroke he was an active man who continued to play tennis and volunteered at the local hospital. According to his wife of 60 years, he was always somewhat stoical and did not show his emotions, but was generally a very happy man. During rehabilitation, he demonstrated frequent agitation and was, therefore, evaluated by a psychiatrist who interviewed him about his mood. Because of his poor communication and frequent stereotypies (he repeatedly said 'OK'), and because the nursing staff stated that J.B. just seemed to be a 'nasty old guy', the psychiatrist did not diagnose depression, but rather prescribed a mild sedative for the agitation. Nursing staff reported a 10 pound weight loss, but viewed it as being due to the poor food at the facility. His sleep was also reported to be poor (he awakened very early each morning and had difficulty falling back to sleep), but the reason for the insomnia was unclear. The speech therapist administered the VAMS to the patient as part of a routine assessment of the response to treatment. The scores are shown in Table 6.2.

**Table 6.2** VAMS scores for J.B.

|         | Afraid | Confused | Sad | Angry | Energetic | Tired | Happy | Tense |
|---------|--------|----------|-----|-------|-----------|-------|-------|-------|
| **Raw**     | 56     | 18       | 69  | 42    | 49        | 48    | 7     | 31    |
| **T-score** | 89     | 53       | 85  | 71    | 42        | 57    | 22    | 59    |

The VAMS indicated that J.B. felt significantly afraid, sad and angry, and had a significantly low level of happiness. Self-reported confusion, energy, fatigue and tension were all within normal limits. At the request of the speech therapist, the psychiatrist was once again consulted and began a trial of paroxetine, a selective serotonin reuptake inhibitor (SSRI). Following 1 month on the SSRI, J.B.'s wife reported that she felt he was feeling much better, in spite of continued significant aphasia and communication difficulties. The VAMS was readministered and showed marked improvement in mood, with all scales falling within normal limits.

## Recommendations for the assessment of mood and depression

The VAMS has been used in a variety of clinical and research settings, in individuals both with and without neurological deficits. The VAMS can be used as a brief screening tool. It can also be used to examine changes in mood over time, such as throughout rehabilitation or therapy, over the course of a treatment or clinical trial, or for studies of mood disorder prevalence in a population (Box 6.3).

### Box 6.3   Appropriate applications of Visual Analog Mood Scales (modified from Stern, 1999)

- Screening for mood disorders by speech-language pathologists and other clinicians to determine if psychiatric/neuropsychiatric consultation is required.
- Assessment of internal mood states in patients who cannot complete more verbally and/or more cognitively demanding instruments.
- Repeated assessment of mood states in clinical practice as a means of monitoring efficacy of an intervention.
- Repeated assessment of mood states in clinical trials research.
- Screening for mood disorder in primary care settings.
- Screening for mood disorder in patients with neurological illness including, but not limited to, dementia, stroke and TBI.

It should be underscored that diagnostic and treatment decisions should not be based solely on the VAMS, or any brief self-report mood scale. Instead, the VAMS should be used as part of a comprehensive analysis of syndromal depression, such as that outlined in Box 6.4. This type of stepwise assessment strategy, including non-verbal methods such as the VAMS, could ultimately improve the reliability and validity of the assessment of specific neurobehavioural syndromes, and contribute to the development of conceptually more useful diagnostic classifications, such as those presented in Box 6.1.

## Box 6.4   Recommendations for the assessment of mood states and neuropsychiatric presentations in patients with acquired communication impairments (modified from Stern, 1996, 1999)

- Obtain a meaningful measure of internal mood state(s) (e.g. VAMS).
- Determine if outward expression of emotion is congruent with internal mood state.
- Do not rely on facial expression, prosodic quality of speech, or displays of laughter or crying, in making a diagnosis.
- Obtain observer reports (from family or nursing staff) regarding apathy.
- Obtain observer reports (from family or other caregivers) of changes in sleep and appetite; if changes exist, determine if they are due to other causes (e.g. medications, acute illness).
- Response to medications (e.g. 'antidepressant') is not equivalent to diagnosis.
- Structural abnormalities on neuroimaging should not guide diagnosis (e.g. left anterior does not *equal* 'depression').

With specific criteria and appropriate assessment tools, this type of classification approach could result in improved understanding of specific neuropathological processes that underlie these distinct presentations. Moreover, clinical trials could be conducted in which differential efficacy of specific treatment modalities could be evaluated, such as: SSRIs for Vegetative Depressive Syndrome, stimulant medications for Apathetic/Abulic Disorder, psychotherapy/counselling for Dysphoric Reaction, and family/caregiver education for Emotional Expression Disorder.

## References

Aitken RC. Measurement of feelings using visual analogue scales. Proc R Soc Med 1969;62: 989–993.

Alderfer BS, Arciniegas DB, Silver JM. Treatment of depression following traumatic brain injury. J Head Trauma Rehabil 2005;20:544–562.

Alexopoulos GS, Abrams RC, Young RC, Shamoian CA. Cornell Scale for Depression in Dementia. Biol Psychiatry 1988;23:271–284.

Alexopoulos GS, Buckwalter K, Olin J, Martinez R, Wainscott C, Krishnan KR. Comorbidity of late life depression: an opportunity for research on mechanisms and treatment. Biol Psychiatry 2002;52:543–558.

Alexopoulos GS, Vrontou C, Kakuma T, Meyers BS, Young RC, Klausner E, Clarkin J. Disability in geriatric depression. Am J Psychiatry 1996;153:877–885.

American Psychiatric Association. Diagnostic and Statistical Manual of Mental Disorders, 4th edn, text revision (DSM-IV-TR). Washington, DC: American Psychiatric Press, Inc., 2000.

Arciniegas DB, Topkoff J, Silver JM. Neuropsychiatric aspects of traumatic brain injury. Curr Treat Options Neurol 2000;2:169–186.

Arruda JE, Stern RA, Legendre SA. Assessment of mood state in patients undergoing electroconvulsive therapy: the utility of visual analog mood scales developed for cognitively impaired patients. Convuls Ther 1996;12:207–212.

Arruda JE, Stern RA, Somerville JA. Measurement of mood states in stroke patients: validation of the visual analog mood scales. Arch Phys Med Rehabil 1999;80:676–680.

Babin PR. Diagnosing depression in persons with brain injuries: a look at theories, the DSM-IV and depression measures. Brain Inj 2003;17:889–900.

Barnes DE, Alexopoulos GS, Lopez OL, Williamson JD, Yaffe K. Depressive symptoms, vascular disease, and mild cognitive impairment: findings from the Cardiovascular Health Study. Arch Gen Psychiatry 2006;63:273–279.

Bergdahl E, Gustavsson JM, Kallin K, von Heideken Wagert P, Lundman B, Bucht G, Gustafson Y. Depression among the oldest old: the Umea 85+ study. Int Psychogeriatr 2005;17:557–575.

Bhalla RK, Papandonatos GD, Stern RA, Ott BR. Alzheimer's disease patients'anxiety prior to and following a standardized on-road driving test. Alzheimer's Dementia 2007;3: 33–39.

Black KJ. Diagnosing depression after stroke. South Med J 1995;88:699–708.

Bowirrat A, Oscar-Berman M, Logroscino G. Association of depression with Alzheimer's disease and vascular dementia in an elderly Arab population of Wadi-Ara, Israel. Int J Geriatr Psychiatry 2006;21:246–251.

Carota A, Staub F, Bogousslavsky J. Emotions, behaviours and mood changes in stroke [Cerebrovascular disease]. Curr Opin Neurol 2002;15:57–69.

Chemerinski E, Levine SR. Neuropsychiatric disorders following vascular brain injury. Mt Sinai J Med 2006;73:1006–1014.

Chemerinski E, Petracca G, Sabe L, Kremer J, Starkstein SE. The specificity of depressive symptoms in patients with Alzheimer's disease. Am J Psychiatry 2001;158:68–72.

Cully JA, Gfeller JD, Heise RA, Ross MJ, Teal CR, Kunik ME. Geriatric depression, medical diagnosis, and functional recovery during acute rehabilitation. Arch Phys Med Rehabil 2005;86:2256–2260.

Cummings JL, Benson DF. Psychological dysfunction accompanying subcortical dementias. Annu Rev Med 1988;39:53–61.

Dam H. Depression in stroke patients 7 years following stroke. Acta Psychiatr Scand 2001;103:287–293.

de Boer AG, van Lanschot JJ, Stalmeier PF, van Sandick JW, Hulscher JB, de Haes JC, Sprangers MA. Is a single-item visual analogue scale as valid, reliable and responsive as multi-item scales in measuring quality of life? Qual Life Res 2004;13:311–320.

Folstein MF, Luria R. Reliability, validity, and clinical application of the Visual Analogue Mood Scale. Psychol Med 1973;3:479–486.

Gainotti G, Azzoni A, Gasparini F, Marra C, Razzano C. Relation of lesion location to verbal and nonverbal mood measures in stroke patients. Stroke 1997;28:2145–2149.

Ganguli M, Du Y, Dodge HH, Ratcliff GG, Chang CC. Depressive symptoms and cognitive decline in late life: a prospective epidemiological study. Arch Gen Psychiatry 2006;63:153–160.

Gelenberg AJ, Hopkins HS. Assessing and treating depression in primary care medicine. Am J Med 2007;120:105–108.

Gordon WA, Hibbard MR, Egelko S, Riley E, Simon D, Diller L, et al. Issues in the diagnosis of post-stroke depression. Rehabil Psychol 1991;36:71–87.

Griffiths MF, Peerson A. Risk factors for chronic insomnia following hospitalization. J Adv Nurs 2005;49:245–253.

Hahn-Barma V, Deweer B, Durr A, Dode C, Feingold J, Pillon B, Agid Y, Brice A, Dubois B. Are cognitive changes the first symptoms of Huntington's disease? A study of gene carriers. J Neurol Neurosurg Psychiatry 1998;64:172–177.

Hamilton M. A rating scale for depression. J Neurol Neurosurg Psychiatry 1960;23:56–62.

Harris Y. Depression as a risk factor for nursing home admission among older individuals. J Am Med Dir Assoc 2007;8:14–20.

Kalpakjian CZ, Lam CS, Leahy BJ. Conceptualization and identification of depression in adults with brain damage by clients and rehabilitation clinical staff. Brain Inj 2002;16:501–507.

Kotila M, Numminen H, Waltimo O, Kaste M. Depression after stroke: results of the FINNSTROKE Study. Stroke 1998;29:368–372.

Kurz AF. Uncommon neurodegenerative causes of dementia. Int Psychogeriatr 2005;17(Suppl. 1):S35–S49.

Lesage AD, Cyr M, Toupin J. Reliable use of the Present State Examination by psychiatric nurses for clinical studies of psychotic and nonpsychotic patients. Acta Psychiatr Scand 1991;83:121–124.

Levin RL, Heller W, Mohanty A, Herrington JD, Miller GA. Cognitive deficits in depression and functional specificity of regional brain activity. Cogn Ther Res 2007;31:211–233.

Lieberman A. Are dementia and depression in Parkinson's disease related? J Neurol Sci 2006;248:138–142.

Lyness JM, Caine ED, Conwell Y, King DA, Cox C. Depressive symptoms, medical illness, and functional status in depressed psychiatric inpatients. Am J Psychiatry 1993;150:910–915.

Lyness JM, Niculescu A, Tu X, Reynolds CF 3rd Caine ED. The relationship of medical comorbidity and depression in older, primary care patients. Psychosomatics 2006;47:435–439.

Marin RS. Differential diagnosis and classification of apathy. Am J Psychiatry 1990;147:22–30.

Marin RS, Wilkosz PA. Disorders of diminished motivation. J Head Trauma Rehabil 2005;20:377–388.

Mirakhur A, Craig D, Hart DJ, McLlroy SP, Passmore AP. Behavioural and psychological syndromes in Alzheimer's disease. Int J Geriatr Psychiatry 2004;19:1035–1039.

Naarding P, de Koning I, dan Kooten F, Dippel DW, Janzing JG, van der Mast RC, Koudstaal PJ. Depression in vascular dementia. Int J Geriatr Psychiatry 2003;18:325–330.

National Center for Health Statistics. Summary Health Statistics for U.S. Adults: National Health Interview Survey, Appendix III, Table IV. Hyattsville, MD: Centers for Disease Control and Prevention, 2005.

Nyenhuis DL, Luchetta T, Yamamoto C, Terrien A, Bernardin L, Rao SM, Garron DC. The development, standardization, and initial validation of the Chicago Multiscale Depression Inventory. J Pers Assess 1998;70:386–401.

Nyenhuis DL, Stern RA, Yamamoto C, Luchetta T, Arruda JE. Standardization and validation of the Visual Analog Mood Scales. Clinical Neurophyschologist 1997;11:407–415.

Paolucci S, Antonucci G, Pratesi L, Traballesi M, Grasso MG, Lubich S. Poststroke depresion and its role in rehabilitation of inpatients. Arch Phys Med Rehab 1999;80:985–990.

Paradiso S, Vaidya J, Tranel D, Kosier T, Robinson RG. Nondysphoric depression following stroke. J Neuropsychiatry Clin Neurosci 2008;20:52–61.

Powell-Tuck J, Hennessy EM. A comparison of mid upper arm circumference, body mass index and weight loss as indices of undernutrition in acutely hospitalized patients. Clin Nutr 2003;22:307–312.

Rigler SK. Management of poststroke depression in older people. Clin Geriatr Med 1999;15:765–783.

Robinson RG, Benson DF. Depression in aphasia patients: Frequency, severity and clinical pathological correlations. Brain Language 1981;14:282–291.

Rogers D, Lees AJ, Smith E, Trimble M, Stern GM. Bradyphrenia in Parkinson's disease and psychomotor retardation in depressive illness. An experimental study. Brain 1987;110:761–776.

Rojo A, Aguilar M, Garolera MT, Cubo E, Navas I, Quintana S. Depression in Parkinson's disease: clinical correlates and outcome. Parkinsonism Relat Disord 2003;10:23–28.

Rosenbek JC, Rodriguez AD, Hieber B, Leon SA, Crucian GP, Ketterson TU, Ciampitti M, Singletary F, Heilman KM, Gonzalez Rothi LJ. Effects of two treatments for aprosodia secondary to acquired brain injury. J Rehabil Res Dev 2006;43:379–90.

Scarmeas N, Hadjigeorgiou GM, Papadimitriou A, Dubois B, Sarazin M, Brandt J, Albert M, Marder K, Bell K, Honig LS, Wegesin D, Stern Y. Motor signs during the course of Alzheimer disease. Neurology 2004;63:975–982.

Scazufca M, Menezes PR, Almeida OP. Caregiver burden in an elderly population with depression in Sao Paulo, Brazil. Soc Psychiatry Psychiatr Epidemiol 2002;37:416–422.

Schrag A. Quality of life and depression in Parkinson's disease. J Neurol Sci 2006;248:151–157.

Schubert DSP, Burns R, Paras W, Sioson E. Increase of medical hospital length of stay by depression in stroke and amputation patients: a pilot study. Psychother Psychosom 1992;57:61–66.

Schwab J, Bialow M, Clemmons R, Martin P, Holzer C. The Beck depression inventory with medical inpatients. Acta Psychiatr Scand 1967;43:255–266.

Simons G, Pasqualini MC, Reddy V, Wood J. Emotional and nonemotional facial expressions in people with Parkinson's disease. J Int Neuropsychol Soc 2004;10:521–535.

Smalbrugge M, Pot AM, Jongenelis L, Gundy CM, Beekman AT, Eefsting JA. The impact of depression and anxiety on well being, disability and use of health care services in nursing home patients. Int J Geriatr Psychiatry 2006;21:325–332.

Starkstein SE, Mizrahi R. Depression in Alzheimer's disease. Expert Rev Neurother 2006;6:887–895.

Starkstein SE, Migliorelli R, Teson A, Petracca G, Chemerinsky E, Manes F, Leiguarda R. Prevalence and clinical correlates of pathological affective display in Alzheimer's disease. J Neurol Neurosurg Psychiatry 1995;59:55–60.

Starkstein SE, Petracca G, Chemerinski E, Kremer J. Syndromic validity of apathy in Alzheimer's disease. Am J Psychiatry 2001;158:872–877.

Steffens DC, Otey E, Alexopoulos GS, Butters MA, Cuthbert B, Ganguli M, et al. Perspectives on depression, mild cognitive impairment, and cognitive decline. Arch Gen Psychiatry 2006;63:130–138.

Stern RA. Assessment of mood states in neurodegenerative disease: methodological issues and diagnostic recommendations. Semin Clin Neuropsychiatry 1996;1:315–324.

Stern RA. Visual Analog Mood Scales: Professional Manual. Odessa, FL: Psychological Assessment Resources, 1997.

Stern RA. Assessment of mood states in aphasia. Semin Speech Lang 1999;20:33–50.

Stern RA, Bachman DL. Depressive symptoms following stroke. Am J Psychiatry 1991;148:351–356.

Stern RA, Bachman DL. Discrepancy between self-report and observer rating of mood in stroke patients: Implications for the differential diagnosis of post-stroke depression [abstract]. J Neuropsych Clin Neurosci 1994;6:319.

Stern RA, Prohaska ML. Neuropsychological evaluation of executive functioning. Am Psychiatr Press Rev Psychiatry 1996;15:243–266.

Stern RA, Arruda JE, Hooper CR, Wolfner GD, Morey CE. Visual Analogue Mood Scales to measure internal mood state in neurologically impaired patients: Description and initial validity evidence. Aphasiology 1997;11:59–71.

Stern RA, Davis JD, Rogers BL, Smith KM, Harrington CJ, Ott BR, Jackson IMD, Prange AJ Jr. Preliminary study of the relationship between thyroid status and cognitive and neuropsychiatric functioning in euthyroid patients with Alzheimer's dementia. Cognit Behav Neurol 2004;17:219–223.

Temple RO, Stern RA, Latham J, Ruffolo JS, Arruda JE, Tremont G. Assessment of mood state in dementia by use of the visual analog mood scales (VAMS). Am J Geriatr Psychiatry 2004;12:527–530.

Townend E, Brady M, McLaughlan K. A systematic evaluation of the adaptation of depression diagnostic methods for stroke survivors who have aphasia. Stroke 2007;38:3076–3083.

Turner-Stokes L, Kalmus M, Hirani D, Clegg F. The Depression Intensity Scale Circles (DISCs): a first evaluation of a simple assessment tool for depression in the context of brain injury. J Neurol Neurosurg Psychiatry 2005;76:1273–1278.

Wang RI, Treul S, Alverno L. A brief self-assessing depression scale. J Clin Pharmacol 1975;15:163–167.

# 7    Interdisciplinary Approaches to the Assessment and Management of Well-Being

**Jane Barton**

Emotional distress following a stroke is extremely common, and this has been discussed at length in earlier chapters. As well as the specific clinical disorders that sometimes occur following stroke, such as clinical depression or clinical anxiety, emotional distress in a more general sense is often present for the majority of patients, and particularly those with communication difficulties. It is, however, important to recognise that emotional distress is often present for many patients who are in hospital, irrespective of whether they have had a stroke or not. Just being unwell and in hospital is very stressful, and can often result in impoverished psychological well-being.

## The experience of being in hospital

There are many accounts in the literature that highlight the psychological experience of patients who are in hospital. There are a number of common themes that tend to emerge with patients, and specifically stroke patients, both with and without communication difficulties.

First, the trauma of being in hospital. Regaining consciousness in hospital can be a terrifying experience as the person starts to realise that they may possibly be unable either to speak or to move, or both, and, indeed, have no understanding of why this might be so. Patients often have no understanding of what stage of recovery they are at, or how long the recovery process is likely to take. Even the process of transferring patients to an alternative ward can be terrifying, particularly as patients often fear the worst, and often fear that this move means that they are going to die.

Second, the thing that patients highlight as being of fundamental importance to them is to be kept informed about what has happened to them, and what is likely to happen to them in the future. They want to be able to understand their condition and the process of recovery, and to be reassured. Perhaps most importantly, patients need to be listened to, and even if they are emotionally upset, the last thing they want is for this distress to be minimised and brushed aside. Again, the process of understanding and of being able to express concerns can be hindered dramatically if the person has communication difficulties as a result of their stroke.

Third, patients often have a range of emotions while in hospital, and these tend to fluctuate over time. Some may feel quite depressed, while others may feel quite anxious. Most are often fearful about the future, wondering what the effect of their stroke will be on their lives and the lives of their families and loved ones. Perhaps one of the most difficult feelings to cope with at this stage is the feeling of no longer being in control, and of losing independence.

Fourth, there are a number of tasks that patients need to undertake at this stage. Perhaps most importantly, patients need to start to try to make sense of what has happened to them, and to understand their medical condition. They need to start to get to know the staff and the hospital system, and to understand what rehabilitation means. Fifth, although most patients are very keen to leave hospital and return home, they are nonetheless often faced with mixed feelings. In particular, patients often fear missing the safety of being in hospital, where they have nurses on hand 24 hours a day to respond to their needs and concerns. This perceived safety net will not be present when they return home. In addition, while in hospital, patients often do not realise the full implications of their disability, and presume that when they return to their own home environment that they will automatically be able to function as well, or nearly as well, as they did prior to the stroke. Returning home can therefore be the point of realisation for patients regarding the extent of their disability, and it is at this point that their mood can often deteriorate significantly.

## The traumatic impact of stroke

Thinking about stroke specifically, it is important to recognise the impact that the stroke has on the person, their life, family and friends, and to understand this within the context of psychological trauma. A stroke often comes completely out of the blue, and inevitably turns the patient's world upside down. The recent shift within the Department of Health to classify stroke as a medical emergency does inevitably highlight the traumatic nature of stroke, rather than seeing it as a health condition of older age. Indeed, from a psychological perspective, there is an emerging body of literature that highlights the traumatic nature of physical illness more generally, and also in relation to stroke (Sembi et al., 1998; Bruggimann et al., 2006), with attention being focused on the development of post-traumatic stress symptoms following the illness event. It is not uncommon to observe signs of psychological trauma in people who have experienced a stroke, either in relation to them psychologically re-experiencing the events of the stroke and possibly having flashbacks in their mind to what actually happened, or alternatively, developing avoidant behaviour regarding anything to do with the stroke or anything that reminds them of having the stroke. There are also a number of models that help in explanation and understanding of the emotional experience of patients going through this process, as patients start to try to understand and make sense of what has happened to them, and start to try to pick up the pieces of their former lives. Moos and Tsu (1977) describe the time phases of a physical illness, and differentiate between the early days and weeks following the event (the crisis phase), the longer-term phase of living with the condition (chronic phase), and the end phase (terminal phase). They describe the psychological (and physical) tasks that patients and families need to undertake in order to cope with the situation that they face. For many stroke patients, the early months following the stroke can therefore be seen as the crisis phase.

Understanding stroke within this context of trauma is important in helping to understand what the emotional experience of patients might be, and what we as professionals might be able to do to help. It is important to recognise that the degree of emotional distress that can occur following a stroke can be huge, although this might not necessarily manifest as an actual clinical disorder. It is nonetheless crucial that this emotional distress is acknowledged and dealt with effectively, by the whole of the multidisciplinary team, as failing to do so will inevitably lead to greater psychological distress in patients, which will in turn have a detrimental effect on the process of rehabilitation and recovery.

## Current practice of mood assessment and management

Assessing and treating mood disorders has traditionally been the work of clinical psychologists and mental health professionals. As such, this has often been a much neglected area of work in general hospital and physical health settings, as very few clinical psychologists tend to be employed to work in these environments. In the case of stroke, an audit by the Royal College of Physicians (2005) identified that only 17% of stroke units in England and Wales had dedicated clinical psychology time, and that on average, only 42% of stroke patients actually had their mood assessed before being discharged from hospital. Despite there being some small areas of good practice where patients' mood is assessed and treated effectively, there is a general recognition that those patients with acquired communication disorders following their stroke will probably be excluded from these formal mood assessments. As well as the lack of trained mental health staff in these environments, there is also the recognition that the standardised mood assessment measures that do exist are not necessarily appropriate for someone who has a communication disorder, either because they are unable to understand or to respond to the verbal questions that are presented. Bennett and Lincoln (2004) have reviewed the use of all mood assessment measures that have been used with stroke. Based on their reliability and validity findings, they have made recommendations for the 'best' assessment tools to use with patients both with and without communication difficulties, in hospital and community rehabilitation settings. There does, however, still appear to be a need for further development of these measures, and this is underway.

In view of this situation described above, where clinical psychologists are employed in stroke unit settings, the role that they often tend to adopt is in terms of training and advice to the rest of the multidisciplinary team (MDT). Thus, the actual routine assessment and management of patients' mood is undertaken by the MDT, with the more complex and challenging cases being picked up by the clinical psychologist or a mental health professional. It is increasingly being recognised that the management of patient well-being is the responsibility of the whole of the MDT, and not just that of the clinical psychologist. Thus, various systems are being set up in stroke units and hospital settings whereby the assessment and routine management of emotional distress following a stroke is undertaken by the nursing, medical, occupational therapy, and speech and language therapy staff, often following training by the clinical psychologist. The role of speech and language therapy staff is particularly crucial here, in advising the MDT on how best to communicate and work with those patients with a communication difficulty (Brumfitt and Barton, 2006).

## Future organisation of mood assessment and management

As discussed above, there is increasing recognition that the assessment and management of patients' mood is not the total responsibility of the clinical psychologist or mental health professional, but rather is the responsibility of the entire multiprofessional team. A number of national policy and guidance documents have recently been published, which highlight the importance of mood assessment and management, and offer some guidance on the roles that MDT professionals can be expected to play. The Royal College of Physicians (2004) published their guidelines on the management of stroke, with (compared to their previous publication in 2000) a larger section being devoted to the psychological management of stroke. In this they clearly highlight the expectation that all stroke patients ought to have their mood assessed, including those patients with communication difficulties, and appropriate treatment be offered while a patient is in hospital. While they recognise that depression is the most common emotional problem following a stroke, they do actually highlight the issue of co-morbidity, and suggest that where one emotional disorder is found to exist, the patient ought to be assessed for other emotional disorders as well. Another recent guideline, this time from the National Institute of Clinical Excellence (NICE, 2004), provides more advice on the actual assessment and management process of depression, in both primary and secondary care. Although this guidance is not specific for use with stroke patients, the high prevalence of depression in stroke patients, particularly those with communication disorders, makes this policy guidance of particular relevance. What NICE (2004) has produced is a stepped model of care, one that clearly sets out the processes that ought to be followed when assessing for depression, both in terms of which professional groups ought to be responsible for the task, and which interventions ought to be offered. The guidelines are relevant to both primary and secondary care (including general hospital settings), and are evidence based in terms of deciding which interventions ought to be offered. The essence of the guideline is that the assessment and management of depression in the first instance is the responsibility of primary care or the general hospital team, with specialist mental health services becoming involved with the more challenging and resistant cases of depression. This model therefore has implications for how depression (and emotional distress) is assessed and managed in stroke patients, and particularly within inpatient hospital settings, as it clearly highlights the role that the different professional groups can make, and does not see the whole task as being within the remit of clinical psychology or mental health services (which are often not present in stroke service settings).

The remainder of this chapter will therefore focus on some aspects of the things that individual members of the MDT can do, and how services need to be organised in order to ensure that we develop an interdisciplinary approach to managing emotional well-being in stroke patients, including those patients with communication difficulties.

## Education and training

### Recognising emotional distress

If the whole of the MDT is going to play an effective role in the assessment and management of patients' mood, then all staff need to receive training in the basic recognition and understanding of emotional disorders such as depression and anxiety, and also how these might be differentiated from the more general experience of emotional distress that has been discussed earlier. Many staff will already have a basic knowledge and understanding of this, but often lack the confidence correctly to identify and name the symptoms that they observe in patients. This is made more difficult in the case of stroke patients, where many of the symptoms observed following a stroke may be similar to symptoms of depression, and differentiating the cause of these can be difficult. This is of course made increasingly difficult when working with patients with post-stroke communication disorders, as the patient may not be able to describe effectively how they are feeling, nor indeed respond to the routine mood assessment questioning.

Bearing in mind that the process of assessing patient mood following a stroke is not an easy task, particularly for those patients with either communication or cognitive difficulties, one of the first things that all MDT staff can do to facilitate this process is to acquaint themselves with the key facts about emotional distress and depression per se, and to increase their understanding of the different ways in which emotional distress can present. It is important to be able to differentiate a patient who may be emotionally distressed because of the traumatic nature of what has happened to them, from someone who has become clinically depressed and is in need of specific targeted treatment for depression.

Many stroke patients describe how they are feeling as being similar to the feelings that people have when they have been bereaved and are grieving. Sharing the idea of this similarity with patients, and describing the psychological processes of grieving, can often be an extremely useful exercise with patients, as patients start to realise that what they are feeling is a 'normal' response to their situation. Models that describe the psychological processes that people go through when they have become bereaved and are grieving can be helpful for patients to start to make sense of their emotional distress and why they might be feeling the way that they are. They are also helpful to staff in enabling them to differentiate what might be a normal process of 'grieving' for the pre-stroke life and identity, from actual clinical disorders. Kubler-Ross (1975) describes one of the most widely used and accepted models of grieving and bereavement, and this is described in Box 7.1.

**Box 7.1   Model of bereavement and grieving (from Kubler-Ross, 1975)**

- Shock
- Denial, disbelief
- Grief, mourning and depression
- Anger
- Adjustment

It is often useful to use this model to have a discussion with patients, to help them understand some of the similarities that can occur between people who have been bereaved and are grieving for a loved one, with themselves who might have lost their own life as they had previously known it before their stroke. Some of these emotional experiences are very similar, and patients can be helped to understand that the strong and intense feelings that they may have are actually 'normal' for the situation that they are in. Normalising these feelings can be crucial for helping patients to understand that they 'are not going mad', something they often fear is happening to them. Patients can start to understand that what they might be experiencing emotionally can be seen as a process, and one that usually, without much targeted intervention, is something they can deal with themselves. Box 7.2 attempts to show how some of the feelings and thoughts that patients experience when emotionally adjusting to their stroke can be similar to the psychological processes of grieving described in the model above. However, it is important to remember that this is not necessarily a linear process for patients, and that they may experience all these thoughts and feelings at various points in their recovery.

### Box 7.2   Model of adjustment

**Shock**
*'I can't believe this has happened'*
*'This has come completely out of the blue'*

**Denial, disbelief**
*'I don't actually believe I've had a stroke, I'll be OK in a few days time'*
*'I'd be alright if I was in my own home'*

**Grief, mourning and depression**
*'I feel so hopeless now that I can't walk . . . my life will never be the same again'*
*'I used to be a lively and energetic person . . . now I feel like hibernating away from everyone . . . my life as I knew it is over'*

**Anger**
*'I wish I'd stopped smoking earlier'*
*'The care that you get in hospital is terrible . . . nobody bothers with you'*

**Adjustment**
*'I can't walk the distances that I used to, but I can use my car to get to the places that I need to now'*
*'I may not be able to talk as well as I did before, but I have found a successful way of communicating with people that I know well'*

Case study 7.1 is an example of a patient who was grieving for their pre-stroke life and identity. In this case the emotional distress that the patient was experiencing was similar to a bereavement reaction, rather than clinical depression.

---

**Case Study 7.1 The bereavement reaction following a stroke**

Alice was a 75-year-old woman who had had a stroke. She had been left with some degree of communication difficulty, which meant that she some-times had word-finding difficulties, and sometimes used the wrong words in conversation. Alice was very distressed about this, and spent much time ruminating about the effect of this on her life. Prior to her stroke, Alice had been very active in her local community, and was in fact the chairperson of her neighbourhood watch group. This inevitably involved her speaking in public. Alice experienced a range of emotions, including sadness at what she believed would be her loss of role in the future. She greatly enjoyed her community activities, and found it difficult to imagine her life without being involved. Over time, Alice came to accept that she was probably always going to have some word-finding difficulties, but once she explained this to her friends and family, and worked out for herself what she felt capable of taking on in the future, she became more positive about her future. She decided to resign as chairperson of her group, but to remain involved and to play an active role. The sadness at her loss of role did not automatically disappear, but Alice felt positive enough to be able to find alternative ways of being involved. It was important for Alice to understand that the sadness that she was experiencing for what she had lost could be seen as similar to someone who is grieving following a bereavement, and it did not necessarily mean that she had become clinically depressed and unable to see a future for herself.

---

Being able to differentiate between other forms of emotional distress and clinical disorders is also important for clinical staff. For example, it may be helpful for staff to understand the difference between depression and post-stroke emotionalism (which is often characterised by uncontrollable crying, but which may not necessarily be associated with low mood). Therefore, having more understanding of the key symptoms of depression and how this may present, will help staff to differentiate clinical mood disorders from the general distress often experienced by the majority of patients in hospital, described above. It is important that staff are aware that depression (and emotional distress) can present in a number of ways. For example, changes in the ways that a person may be behaving or feeling physically. Drawing on a range of these different types of symptoms, and observations of behaviour, can be crucial in helping correctly to identify emotional disorders in patients with communication difficulties, as reliance on verbal descriptions by the patient may be more limiting. The clinical psychologist can play a crucial role here, in educating staff more reliably to identify and name emotional disorders when they observe symptoms as part of their routine daily care, and particularly so when patients, due to their communication difficulties, cannot reliably describe how they are feeling. Table 7.1 lists the most common signs and symptoms of depression and anxiety, which are crucial for staff to be aware of. Charts detailing these symptoms can be posted on the walls of wards, not only to remind staff of the signs and symptoms to look out for and act upon, but also to highlight the prevalence of depression and mood disorders to patients and families who are visiting, so that they too can play a role in recognising and correctly identifying if their loved one is in need of professional intervention.

**Table 7.1** Common signs and symptoms of depression and anxiety.

| | Depression: signs and symptoms | Anxiety: signs and symptoms |
|---|---|---|
| Thoughts and feelings | I can't cope | Constant worrying |
| | I am to blame | What if this happens again? |
| | Hopelessness | What will people think of me? |
| | Negative outlook (self and world) | What if I can't cope? |
| | Sadness | How will I manage at home? |
| | Suicidal thoughts | How will I be able to talk to my |
| | Tearfulness | family? |
| Behaviour | Social withdrawal | Social withdrawal |
| | Apathy | Apathy |
| | Inactivity | Increased activity |
| | Avoidance | Ritualised behaviours |
| Physical | Poor concentration | Palpitations |
| | Poor memory | Chest pain |
| | Fatigue and listlessness | Butterflies in stomach |
| | Disturbed appetite | Dry mouth |
| | Disturbed sleep | Sweating |
| | | Breathlessness |

In addition to increasing awareness of the different ways in which depression and emotional distress can manifest, staff ought to be aware of some of the key factors that are known to place certain patients at a greater risk of developing depression than others. For example, having a past history of diagnosed depression, or a family history of depression, is likely to make a person more vulnerable to developing depression in the future. In addition, having little social support or being socially isolated can also place a person at a greater risk of developing depression. Again, having this knowledge and awareness can be extremely helpful for staff in monitoring the emotional state of patients, and increasing their confidence to be able to correctly identify those patients who appear to be at greater risk of developing clinical depression, particularly where patients may not be able to report this themselves. Case study 7.2 is an example of a patient who had communication difficulties, and was unable to let the staff know how he was feeling.

---

**Case Study 7.2 Assessing the risk of depression with impaired communication**

John was an 82-year-old man who was on the stroke rehabilitation unit. Although he was able to understand some of what people were saying to him, his communication difficulties meant he was unable to express how he was feeling. The nurses started to notice that John was not always eating his meals, and sometimes even refused them altogether. The physiotherapist also reported that although John did attend their therapy sessions, it seemed as if he was lacking in energy, and finding it difficult to focus on the task in hand. Discussion at the weekly MDT meeting revealed that John did in fact have a past history of depression, and that he had been taking antidepressant medication for many years in his earlier life. However, his mood had been stable prior to admission to hospital. It was also highlighted that John had been recently bereaved—his wife had died 18 months previously. These factors alerted the MDT to consider that John might again be feeling depressed, and that because of his communication difficulties no formal mood screening had been undertaken. The speech and language therapist spent her next session with John looking at different pictures of emotional expressions, and John very clearly highlighted the images depicting expressions of sadness and hopelessness as reflecting how he was feeling. Although many of the signs and symptoms that staff noticed about John were clearly signs of depression, it was only when factors associated with John's life prior to his stroke were taken into consideration that staff were able to understand this as being depression.

---

As well as gaining more understanding of how depression and anxiety might present, becoming more familiar with the way in which psychological symptoms of trauma often present can also be very helpful. Typically, the basic symptoms observed in someone who is experiencing post-traumatic stress include persistent re-experiencing through images, nightmares and flashbacks; along with avoidance of stimuli associated with the trauma (APA, 1994). In addition, there will be persistent symptoms of increased arousal and numbing of general responsiveness (APA, 1994).

Case study 7.3 is an example of a stroke patient who was displaying symptoms of trauma following their stroke.

---

**Case Study 7.3 Symptoms of post-traumatic stress following a stroke**

Joe was a 65-year-old man who had his stroke while he was up a ladder mending the roof of his house. He did not lose consciousness, but became physically paralysed and was unable to move. He was eventually lifted from the roof of his house by the fire brigade, but all the time Joe was fearing for his life. During his recovery in hospital, and for a few months after returning home, Joe would experience flashbacks about being on the roof of the house, and actually re-experienced the traumatic feelings of fear that he had at the time. He did not have control over these flashbacks, which tended to occur as intrusive memories that would happen spontaneously. It felt to Joe as if he was re-experiencing the stroke all over again, and this was obviously extremely distressing for him. It was explained to Joe that these flashbacks were a symptom of post-traumatic stress, which can occur when someone has been involved in a traumatic incident where there has been a threat to their life, and Joe was given some strategies to help him deal with this.

## Increasing staff confidence

Staff belonging to a MDT are becoming increasingly knowledgeable about recognising depression in their patients, yet they do not always have the confidence to know what to do once they have identified it. The majority of staff often feel that they do not have the appropriate skills and expertise to be able to work with patients who are emotionally distressed, and who may also have a communication difficulty. This often leads to staff avoiding having interactions with patients, for fear that they will not know how to handle the patient's distress, nor indeed be able to communicate effectively with patients who are unable to talk. They often fear that if they were to start a 'conversation' with a patient about how they are feeling, then this might open the flood gates, and the patient might become so distressed that the member of staff becomes overwhelmed and does not know how to manage the situation. Training in how to have meaningful interactions with patients, and to be able to respond to their emotional distress, is fundamentally important and is something that can be undertaken by the clinical psychologist, often in conjunction with the speech and language therapist. Having some tips on knowing what to do if a patient becomes upset or distressed, as well as tips on having 'conversations' with patients with communication difficulties, is fundamentally important in helping staff to feel more confident and competent about having interactions with and responding to patients.

Training staff in basic counselling skills is useful in this context. The majority of staff will inevitably already possess these basic counselling skills, which they will have picked up and developed throughout their caring career. We are not talking here about formal counselling methods, but rather the general principles of a counselling interaction, and those which we know are crucial to patient well-being. By this I mean the basic counselling skills, which include: empathy, active listening, reflecting back and reformulation. Box 7.3 gives more information on these useful skills.

### Box 7.3   Basic counselling skills

- *Empathy*—This involves trying to *feel with*, rather than to *feel for* the patient. It means that you have understood the feelings that the patient is experiencing, and that you have communicated this understanding to the patient. It involves trying to see the world through the eyes of the patient, while at the same time not losing a sense of objectivity or introducing bias.
- *Reflecting back and reformulation*—This involves trying to look for the basic message that the patient is trying to convey, and trying to restate or summarise this basic message in your own words. This is effective because: it lets the patient know that you are trying to understand them; it checks that you have understood what the patient is trying to

convey; it helps the patient to clarify what they are actually thinking about, and how they are feeling; and it helps the patient to continue.

- *Active listening*—This is a skill, and is hard work! It involves a combination of many skills, including: non-verbal communication, for example holding eye contact, or keeping an open posture; verbal communication, for example, responding to the patient by reflecting and reformulating, using phrases like 'I see what you mean', and avoiding sending discouraging messages by interrupting or changing the subject.

Many staff do not feel confident or competent to explore feelings, largely because they fear that the situation may escalate out of control. This increases anxiety in staff members. Having a few basic tips on how to respond to patients who might be distressed can be useful for staff to follow. Box 7.4 gives a summary of some pointers that can be helpful.

### Box 7.4 Tips on how to respond to emotional distress

1. Listening to the patient is perhaps the most crucial skill. This is not always easy, however, but using a combination of verbal and non-verbal methods of communication this can be made easier.
2. Let the patient know that you have heard what they are 'saying' and that you have understood. If you have not understood what the patient is trying to communicate to you, it is important to acknowledge this with the patient, and suggest that you will need to do some more exploration of what the problem is.
3. Try to concentrate on what the patient is trying to communicate to you. Focus on how the patient is behaving, as well as what they are saying.
4. Remember that if a patient is distressed or is crying, it is important for the member of staff to acknowledge this distress with the patient, and not to avoid it or shy away from it. The last thing that patients want to hear when they are upset is that 'everything will be alright!' Of course patients do want reassurance, but they also want to have their distress acknowledged and validated.
5. Remember to make eye contact with the patient, and try to keep an open body posture, so that the patient knows that you are interested in what they are trying to communicate to you.

However, there are times when patients may display very extreme forms of emotions, and may become angry. This is not uncommon when patients are undergoing medical traumas, and are perhaps not feeling very well. Again, staff can respond appropriately and effectively in these situations, using their basic counselling skills, which inevitably will have a positive impact on patient well-being. Box 7.5 lists a number of points to take into consideration when a patient becomes angry.

**Box 7.5   Tips on dealing with extremes of emotion**

1. Try to stay calm, at least on the outside.
2. Do not argue with the patient.
3. Try not to become agitated or let the patient know that you are feeling uncomfortable.
4. Continue to speak at your usual pace and volume, without your voice becoming raised.
5. It is advisable to acknowledge openly that the person is angry, and to gently enquire why. This can often take the heat out of the situation, but can also leave you feeling both emotionally and physically drained.
6. After the event it is often helpful to acknowledge your own feelings here, and probably best to find a colleague to talk to.

Training programmes can be developed for staff, to help them to increase their confidence to work with patients with emotional and communication difficulties. One such programme was developed in our stroke service, in a large teaching hospital in the north of England, and was run by the clinical psychologist, speech and language therapist, and occupational therapist. The training runs over two days, and focuses on increasing awareness and understanding of psychological (emotional and cognitive) and communication difficulties following stroke, as well as developing skills to work with these. A series of homework assignments are undertaken by participants, where they have the opportunity to develop and practise the skills that they have learned in their actual work environments. Pre- and post-course evaluations are made of participants' knowledge, as well as confidence to undertake this work. The training is open to all professions within the MDT, both qualified and unqualified staff. Case study 7.4 describes the experience of a nurse who attended the training, and the impact that this had on her clinical practice in addressing the emotional needs of patients.

---

**Case Study 7.4  Impact of staff awareness training**

Kate had been qualified as a nurse for 7 years. At the start of the training course she described that she did not feel confident to talk to patients if they were visibly distressed, and particularly if they had communication difficulties, as she feared that if she became involved she would either not be able to understand what patients were trying to communicate to her, or that the patients' distress might escalate and she would become helpless and overwhelmed. Through undertaking the homework assignments, Kate reported that she had 'practised' having a 'conversation' with a patient with aphasia, and who was obviously distressed about something. She reported that she remembered the tips from the course on the importance of just listening to, and being able to stay with a person's distress, as well as using aspects of supported conversation (e.g. using paper, pens and pictures). The outcome of the course for Kate was that she felt more confident and competent to have 'conversations' with patients who were distressed, and she felt more comfortable to be able just to listen to what the patient was saying, rather than feeling as if she had to solve the problem for the patient. She made a resolution to herself that she would start routinely to ask patients how they were feeling, and allocate some time to be able to listen to their responses, something that she had previously avoided doing, and perhaps most importantly to include patients with communication difficulties in this promise.

---

## Knowing which assessment tools to use

As discussed earlier, when it comes to the assessment of depression, it is not a case of 'one size fits all', and knowing which mood assessment tools are the most appropriate to use, and with which patient, can be difficult, particularly where the patient may have either cognitive or communication difficulties. Based on the review of assessment measures conducted by Bennett and Lincoln (2004), identifying the 'best' assessment tool for use with patients is crucial. Speech and language therapists can play a vital role here, often in advising the rest of the MDT (or specifically the member of staff who is going to undertake the formal mood assessment) as to the patient's degree of communication disability, and their understanding of verbally presented information (Brumfitt and Barton, 2006). As the different assessment tools require varying levels of language comprehension, the speech and language therapist is perhaps best placed to advise on and select the most appropriate assessment tool. An example of how this can be operationalised is as follows, using a hierarchical system that can be developed based on the person's degree of aphasia. For those patients with a mild aphasia, it may be appropriate to use the routine mood assessment measures that are used in the service with all patients, for example, the Hospital Anxiety and Depression Scale (HADS) (Zigmond and Snaith, 1983). However, for patients with a moderate degree of aphasia, where their ability to understand and respond to verbally presented information is somewhat impaired, an alternative, visually presented assessment measure of mood may be appropriate, such as the Depression Intensity Scale Circles (DISCs) (Turner-Stokes, Kalmus, Hirani and Clegg, 2005). For those patients with a more severe degree of aphasia, however, an alternative type of assessment measure based on staff (and/or family) observations of the patient over a period of time might be most appropriate to use, such as the Stroke Aphasic Depression Questionnaire (SADQ-10) (Sutcliffe and Lincoln, 1998). The speech and language therapist's evaluation of the patient's level of communication disability will be vital here in helping to determine which is the most appropriate assessment measure to use. It is sometimes necessary to use a combination of assessment tools, and of course to review the outcomes over time. Training on how to administer and interpret the results from the screening tools is vitally important, and this has been discussed earlier. It is important, however, to remember that the screening measures that are often used offer only an indication of a patient's emotional state. They do not actually diagnose the presence of depression in a patient. Further assessment following the screening assessment is important for a diagnosis of depression to be made.

Informal assessment of mood and emotional distress can often play as a crucial a role as the more formal assessment processes that are in place. Therapists are often best placed to observe and comment on patients' behaviour, largely in terms of how the patient presents in the therapy sessions. For example, changes in how well the patient may be engaging in their physiotherapy or occupational therapy, may be crucial information in helping to understand how the patient is feeling. It is not uncommon for therapists to observe changes in patients' behaviour that could reflect underlying changes in their mood. For example, behaviours of concern would include withdrawing from their therapy sessions, or not wanting to participate in active rehabilitation. However, understanding why this might be the case can provide useful information as to how the patient is actually feeling. The following case study is a useful illustration of how such information gained through observation in therapy sessions can play a crucial part on the overall assessment of a patient's mood. Case study 7.5 describes the case of a stroke patient whose change in behaviour alerted staff to further explore the patient's feelings.

---

**Case Study 7.5 The importance of observations by staff members**

Jack was a 79-year-old man who was undergoing rehabilitation following his stroke. He had a range of residual impairments, including mild aphasia, and difficulties in walking. Jack was always very keen to participate in therapy in hospital, and showed no obvious signs of depression. Staff were pleased with the progress that Jack was making. After a while, the physiotherapist noticed that Jack was not as engaged with his rehab as he had previously been, and there were a couple of times when he had refused to go to therapy at all. The therapist commented to Jack about what they had observed. Using a combination of talking, pictures and other aspects of supported conversation, Jack was able to describe that he had become disillusioned with his therapy, and felt that he was not making as much progress as he had expected. He felt that he could not see the point of putting in all the hard work that he had, if he could not see that he was making sufficient progress. He reported feeling low and unmotivated, and had difficulty seeing a positive future. The therapist explained to Jack that he was making progress, and the reason why he was perhaps not able to see this was because he was feeling depressed. The therapist and the rest of the MDT were then able to look at possible interventions to address Jack's depression.

## Psychologically sophisticated environments

It is important to consider the context in which emotional care is delivered. Whereas many health service settings would argue that they provide good psychological care, there is a general feeling that what care is offered is often patchy and inconsistent. Nichols (1993, 2005) has written extensively about this, and argues that what is required is a scheme of delivering psychological care that can match the level of physical care that is given. He argues that in order to provide good psychological care, this needs to consist of more than being a caring professional who helps a patient with their impairments as and when they arise. Environments that are psychologically sophisticated deliver emotional care in a systematic and routine way. The question that he asks is: can the service be confident that the psychological care that they deliver is both timely and meaningful, and can they be confident that this will be available for all patients? He thus argues that a system of psychological care needs to be in place that is structured, routine and timely for all patients, and that this is fundamentally crucial for addressing the emotional well-being of patients. Box 7.6 lists a number of questions posed by Nichols that services can ask of themselves, in order to assess the sophistication of psychological care that they deliver.

**Box 7.6   Questions to assess the sophistication of psychological care (Nichols, 1993)**

- Are the nurses and therapists trained?
- Is there an explicit scheme of psychological care?
- Is there an allocation of 'psychological duties' to staff? Is it systematic?
- Are there prepared materials?
- Are there records of psychological and educational interventions?
- Is there a guarantee of psychological care for all clients and/or caregivers?
- Do medical staff coordinate their work with the psychological interventions?

Reproduced with permission of Springer Publications.

Drawing on the work and ideas of Nichols discussed above, if the MDT is to become successful in ensuring that all patients have their mood assessed and monitored while in hospital, then a structure needs to be put into place to make this happen. One way that this can be achieved is to introduce the idea of having care plans for each patient, which are specifically devoted to the emotional and psychological care of the patient. The use of care plans is well established within physical health (and particularly nursing) settings, and these primarily tend to focus on monitoring aspects of physical care. The introduction of care plans that focus on the psychological needs of patients can be one measure to help ensure that patient mood is systematically and routinely assessed and monitored for each patient while they are in hospital. At the same time it also clearly highlights that this is the responsibility of the whole MDT, not just the task of the psychologist or mental health worker.

Key principles to consider when designing care plans that aim to make psychological care both routine and systematic are as follows:

1. The emotional care plans ought to be inserted into the patient's notes routinely at the start of treatment.
2. All patients (including those with communication difficulties) will have an emotional care plan, regardless of whether or not they appear to be suffering with their mood. This is partly to take account of the fact that impairments with mood following a stroke can fluctuate. Some patients may not show any signs or symptoms of low mood at one point in time, but this can change very quickly, and thus needs to be continually monitored.
3. A system of key workers could be established, whereby one person is responsible for ensuring that the emotional care plans are completed appropriately, and any necessary action is taken. However, it should not be the total responsibility of the key worker to provide all the emotional care for the patient, but rather the responsibility of the whole MDT to deliver this care by incorporating this into the routine aspects of their work.
4. In order to ensure that routine emotional care is provided, a step by step approach ought to be detailed on the care plan, in order for the key worker to follow a prescribed set of steps. This can help to standardise the process, and ensure that all patients are receiving the same standard of care and monitoring.
5. Options can be provided on the care plan as to the most appropriate screening tools to use, depending on whether or not the patient has any communication difficulties, and if so, the extent of these difficulties. These options ought to be based on the best available evidence from within the literature, discussed earlier.
6. Any action to be taken, based on the results of the assessment measures, must be clearly identified on the care plan, and some guidance given as to who is responsible for doing this. For example, if a comprehensive

diagnostic assessment interview is requested, it should state by whom (e.g. medical staff), and the outcome clearly documented.

7. A range of possible interventions to address emotional distress can be listed, which are evidence based, as detailed for example in the NICE guidelines for the management of depression. These can then be tailored to what the service can actually offer, largely in terms of what skills and resources are available to the team.

8. Perhaps most importantly, the process of developing the emotional care plan ought to involve the whole MDT. This can help to ensure that all members of staff feel some ownership of the process, and as a result are more likely to engage with the process.

## Conclusions

There has been a significant increase in recognition within stroke services that much emotional distress can occur following a stroke, particularly for those patients with communication difficulties. In recent years various national guidelines and directives have been published, which offer some guidance as to the best forms of assessment and management of mood disorders in general, and in stroke specifically. What this chapter has attempted to highlight is the role of the multidisciplinary stroke team in this assessment and management process. While this work has traditionally been within the remit of clinical psychologists and mental health workers, there is now a greater acceptance that the *routine* assessment and management of mood disorders ought to be undertaken by the MDT, with specialist mental health trained workers becoming involved with more chronic and challenging cases, as well as the basic training of the MDT. Some examples have been offered within this chapter of how such service provision might be organised, and the roles that the various members of the MDT might undertake in this process. As might be expected, the role of the speech and language therapist is crucial in facilitating this process for those patients with communication difficulties following their stroke.

## References

American Psychiatric Association. Diagnostic and Statistical Manual of Mental Disorders, 4th edn. Washington DC: APA, 1994.

Bennett HE, Lincoln N. Screening for Depression after Stroke. London: The Stroke Association, 2004.

Bruggimann L, Annoni JM, Staub F, von Steinbuchel N, van der Linden M, Bogousslavsky J. Chronic posttraumatic stress symptoms after nonsevere stroke. Neurology 2006;66:513–516.

Brumfitt S, Barton J. Evaluating well-being in people with aphasia using speech therapy and clinical psychology. Int J Ther Rehab 2006;13:305–310.

Kubler-Ross E. Death: The Final Stage of Growth. New York: Prentice Hall, 1975.

Moos RH, Tsu VD. The crisis of physical illness. In: Moos RH (ed.) Coping with Physical Illness. New York: Plenum, 1977.

National Institute for Clinical Excellence. Management of Depression in Primary and Secondary Care. Clinical Guideline 23. London: NICE, 2004.

Nichols KA. Psychological Care in Physical Illness, 2nd edn. London: Chapman & Hall, 1993.

Nichols K. Why is psychology still failing the average patient? Psychologist 2005;18:26–27.

Royal College of Physicians. National Clinical Guidelines for Stroke, 2nd edn. London: RCP, 2004.

Royal College of Physicians. National Sentinel Audit of Stroke. London: RCP, 2005.

Sembi S, Tarrier N, O'Neill P, Burns A, Farragher B. Does post traumatic stress disorder occur after stroke: A preliminary study. Int J Geriatric Psychiatry 1998;13:315–322.

Sutcliffe L, Lincoln N. The assessment of depression in aphasic stroke patients. The development of the Stroke Aphasia Depression Scale. Clin Rehabil 1998;12:506–513.

Turner-Stokes L, Kalmus M, Hirani D, Clegg F. The Depression Intensity Scale Circles (DISCs): Initial evaluation of a simple assessment tool for depression in the context of brain injury. J Neurol Neurosurg Psych 2005;76:1273–1278.

Zigmond AS, Snaith RP. The hospital anxiety and depression scale. Acta Psychiatr Scand 1983;67:361–370.

# 8 Psychological Approaches to Working with People in the Early Stages of Recovery

## Shonagh Scott and Jane Barton

Authors in the earlier chapters of this book have discussed in detail the common psychological and emotional reactions that people experience following a stroke. We know that 20–50% of patients will be clinically depressed; 20–40% will be affected by anxiety; and at least 35% of those who survive a stroke will have significant intellectual impairment. In addition, people may experience post-stroke emotionalism and difficulties adjusting emotionally to the changes precipitated by the stroke. The literature also suggests that people with aphasia may be at an increased risk of suffering from depression following a stroke.

## Understanding the emotional impact of stroke

One framework that helps us to understand the emotional aspects of coping with a stroke is in terms of time phases in a chronic illness. Moos and Tsu (1977) describe the developmental time phases of a chronic illness as an ongoing process with landmarks, transitions and changing demands. They describe three time phases, and the adaptive tasks which the patient and their families need to undertake at each:

1. *Crisis phase*—acute phase following the onset of the illness. The patient and their family need to:
   - create a meaning for the illness event that maximises a preservation of a sense of mastery and competency;
   - grieve for the loss of the pre-illness family identity;
   - move towards a position of acceptance of permanent change while maintaining a sense of continuity between the past and the future;
   - pull together to undergo short-term crisis reorganisation;
   - in the face of uncertainty, develop a system of flexibility towards future goals.
2. *Chronic phase*—the day-to-day living with chronic illness. A key task of this period is the maintenance by the patient and their family of a

semblance of normal life under the 'abnormal' presence of a chronic illness and heightened uncertainty. In addition, the maintenance of maximal autonomy for all family members in the face of the pull towards mutual dependency and caretaking.
3. *Terminal phase*—where the inevitability of death becomes apparent and dominates family life. Issues surrounding this phase include: separation, death, grief, resolution of mourning and resolution of 'normal' family life beyond this loss.

Following the immediate medical emergency of the stroke, patients are transferred from acute neurology wards when they become medically stable and it is thought that they can benefit from rehabilitation. Both patients and families at this point experience a range of emotions. There is often the feeling of shock and disbelief at what has happened, and in some cases a sense of denial. Anxiety is often the most significant problem at this stage. Not only is the patient concerned and worried about their future, both in terms of how they are going to manage, and in terms of their health, but so are their families and partners. Partners at this stage will perhaps not see themselves as carers, but rather relatives of someone who is ill in hospital. It is only as the process of rehabilitation proceeds that this realisation that they are likely to become carers sets in. Both the patient and the family are at the very early stage of adjustment. In terms of Moos and Tsu's classification, in the acute crisis phase patients and families may be initially numb with shock and disbelief at what has happened and need to repeat their 'stroke story' to help accept the reality of what has happened. The importance of 'telling your story' is discussed in detail later in this chapter.

In Sheffield many patients are discharged from hospital into the Community Rehabilitation Teams (CRT), where they continue to have rehabilitation in their own homes for up to 12 weeks. Being discharged from hospital and coming home will often raise a number of worries and concerns for both the patient and their family. In terms of Moos and Tsu's classification, the patient and family are perhaps still in the crisis phase of coping with and managing their stroke. Major anxieties are often around how everyone will cope, what changes will need to take place in order to adapt and what the future is likely to hold. It is probably only at this stage that the partner begins fully to realise the situation, and to take on the role of becoming a carer.

During this period of rehabilitation, recovery will take place, and patients and families tend to make the necessary physical and emotional adjustments to live with the aftermath of the stroke. Coping now is perhaps seen more in terms of the chronic day-to-day living with the illness. However, in some instances, the realisation for either the patient or their family that a full recovery may not take place, and that residual disabilities may remain, can lead to intense feelings of loss and depression.

Patients and families are often heard to ask the question 'Is this as good as it will get?', as recovery gains that they had hoped for may not have actually been achieved. There can be ongoing tension between hope for complete recovery and the reality of accepting limits and losses of ability and roles.

## Psychological care vs psychological intervention

The number of clinical psychologists working in stroke services falls far short of the number ideally recommended, and they tend therefore to be a scarce resource. Recent Royal College of Physician Guidelines (Royal College of Physicians, 2004) for stroke recommended that clinical psychologists should be members of the specialist stroke team. However, the recent Sentinel Audit of stroke services in England and Wales (Royal College of Physicians, 2004) identified that only 17% of stroke services had clinical psychology input. This discrepancy between recommendation and reality leads to the important question of who else might be able to perform basic psychological assessment and interventions? Nichols (2003, 2005) provides a model for understanding levels of psychological care as distinct from psychological treatments (such as cognitive behavioural therapy). The model is outlined in Table 8.1. He describes psychological care as 'an approach to looking after the ill and injured that can be integrated with nursing or the various therapies to provide an organised and practical psychological content to overall care.' The content of psychological care utilises skills that are already in existence within the multidisciplinary team and can be implemented by all members of the team including doctors, nurses, therapists and unqualified care staff. These include regular monitoring of psychological state, providing information, emotional care and, if necessary, initiating referral to a clinical psychologist for psychological therapy. Psychological care should be provided by all professionals who have direct contact with the patient and should be a routine, integral part of caring for the patient in a holistic way. Indeed, Nichols goes so far as to assert that 'for a health care professional to walk away from a patient with

**Table 8.1** The components of psychological care (from Nichols, 2003).

| Level 1 (awareness) | Awareness of psychological issues |
| --- | --- |
| | Patient-centred listening |
| | Patient-centred communication |
| | Awareness of the patient's psychological state and relevant action |
| Level 2 (intervention) | Monitoring the patient's psychological state with records kept |
| | Informational and educational care |
| | Emotional care |
| | Counselling care |
| | Support/advocacy/referral |
| Level 3 (therapy) | Psychological therapy |

no knowledge of how they are coping or whether they are confused or in distress is the opposite of holistic care. In my view it is very unprofessional.' Most of the interventions outlined in this chapter will fall into the category of psychological care rather than psychological intervention, in order to reflect that it is likely to be members of the multidisciplinary team, other than the clinical psychologist, who will deliver the care.

## Addressing psychological needs and working with emotions

Before we discuss specific interventions it may be helpful to remind ourselves of some of the basic general counselling skills, such as empathy, reformulating and active listening, that should underpin any interaction with patients. The acute physical event of a stroke cannot be separated from the person with the stroke, and therefore the psychological aspects of care cannot be separated from the physical aspects of care: the two are inextricably linked. It is important for us to remind ourselves that the patient in front of us existed before the stroke and for us to try to have some idea as to what that pre-stroke individual was like. An intervention as simple as spending some time with a patient and their family to find out what their lives were like before the stroke and how their lives have changed since, not only can provide a sense of the 'whole person' but also gives us some ideas as to possible goals for rehabilitation. All too often as professionals we can become focused on the disability or impairment that needs treating rather than trying to bear the whole person in mind. If as professionals we just focus on physical symptoms alone and then give advice, it is likely that the patient will not be receptive to what we have to say. This is because the patient may be too preoccupied with undisclosed thoughts and feelings to concentrate on what we are saying. The presence of strong emotions that are not identified or acknowledged will prevent open communication from taking place. It is only when we have understood the patients' emotions and concerns that we can move on to explore the best way to help. Professionals can, understandably, put up barriers to exploring emotions with patients. Staff often feel that if they start trying to explore emotions and feelings they will open the floodgates and the outpouring of emotions will overwhelm them. Staff may develop a protective shell to shield themselves from becoming upset, and develop ways of distancing themselves from having to deal with feelings (e.g. 'I'm just a nurse, you'll have to ask the doctor about that' or 'I'll ask the psychologist to come and speak to you'). As well as feeling potentially overwhelmed by emotions, staff may feel anxious because dealing with strong feelings in others can arouse strong feelings in ourselves. Our behaviour often changes, and we become more concerned with monitoring our own internal state rather than attending to the patient. These changes in our own behaviour are often spotted by the patient, who reacts to them, perhaps by becoming ill at ease, which in turn may make us more anxious and so a vicious circle is formed.

By utilising our basic general counselling skills we can feel more confident in addressing psychological need and discussing emotions with patients. One of the most important skills is that of *active listening*. Active listening involves non-verbal communication, such as making eye contact with the patient when they are talking and maintaining an open body posture to indicate that you are interested in what they are saying, rather than standing at the foot of the bed with your arms crossed. Active listening also includes verbal behaviour such as responding to the patient by reflecting back to them what they have been saying and using comments like 'I see what you mean' or 'I follow you', which signals that you are listening and encouraging the patient to continue. It is important when actively listening to a patient not to send discouraging messages by interrupting them, changing the subject, not acknowledging what the person has said, or by interrogating them rather than reflecting and summarising. Concentrate on the patient and try to understand what they are saying and feeling, so that you can respond appropriately.

This leads us on to the skill of *empathy*, which is an important means for understanding patients and letting them know that they are understood. It involves trying to see the world through their eyes, but without losing your sense of objectivity, and requires a certain amount of identification with what the person is feeling and saying while retaining a degree of detachment so you do not become immersed and biased. Sympathy and compassion focus on your feelings rather than the patient's feelings. Empathy is trying to feel with the patient, rather then trying to feel for the patient. It means that you have understood the feelings that the patient is experiencing, and that you have communicated this understanding to the patient. Trying to rephrase or to *reformulate* what a patient has said is an important way of developing an empathic understanding. When reformulating it is useful to look for the basic message in what the patient is trying to communicate and to restate or summarise the basic message back to the patient in your own words. When reformulating it is important to do this in a tentative, wondering way, rather than an absolute way, as this allows the patient to confirm your understanding or correct if necessary. Reformulating is an effective counselling skill because it communicates to the patient that you are trying to understand them and it helps to test your understanding of what the patient has said. It also helps the patient to clarify what they think and feel and focuses attention on particular aspects of what was said and encourages the patient to continue.

## Psychological care and interventions

The remainder of this chapter focuses on specific examples of psychological care and intervention, many of which have been developed by the authors and other colleagues in Sheffield. Psychological interventions following stroke can be either indirect or direct interventions. Indirect interventions can be provided by any member of the multidisciplinary team, whereas direct interventions tend to be provided directly by, or under the close supervision of, clinical psychologists. Indirect interventions focus on overall psychological well-being and the 'normal' process of adjustment to stroke, whereas direct interventions focus on more significant mental health difficulties, for example depression, anxiety, trauma or problems with adjustment to the stroke.

### Indirect interventions

### Providing information

In the very early days following a stroke, depending on the medical condition of the person, it is likely to be the family that requires information from professionals about medical investigations and prognosis. At this stage the role of the Family Support Worker can be invaluable. The Family Support Service is run by the Stroke Association, and workers can visit the patient in hospital and at home after discharge. Their role is to look at the needs of the person and their family, and give advice, emotional support and information to help people understand the effects of the stroke. They can also link people into local services and groups and help them liaise with health services, social services and voluntary organisations.

Once medically stable, the person who has had the stroke will need information about what has happened to them; how long they can expect to stay in hospital and what will happen to them whilst in hospital; when they can expect to be discharged; and post-discharge care plans. The Stroke Association provides excellent leaflets about all aspects of stroke, including *Psychological Effects of Stroke*, *Cognitive Problems after Stroke*, and *Communication Problems after Stroke*. The information needs to be provided at the right time for the patient to be able to absorb it—there would be little point in providing someone with information about driving after a stroke if their main concern was their speech and language difficulties. For people with aphasia the information must be aphasia friendly. Later in this chapter an aphasia friendly tool for facilitating rehabilitation will be discussed in detail. The aim of providing information to patients and their families is to reduce anxiety and to increase the person's sense of control over the situation and their rehabilitation. Often the same information needs to be provided on several occasions before patients are finally able to 'hear' it and take it on board. A recent study by the Stroke Association (2006) looked at the information patients were provided with on discharge from hospital. They found that vital health information on how to prevent further strokes as well as signposting to relevant rehabilitation services, access to benefits, and even details on prescribed medication was severely lacking. This lack of information left patients and their families feeling abandoned and lost after leaving hospital. Unfortunately, even when people were given information on discharge it was often in a format that they struggled to understand due to cognitive or sensory impairments or speech and language problems. Only half of the stroke patients in the study said that they were able to understand the information they were given in hospital about their condition.

In one of the acute hospitals in Sheffield the stroke unit holds a weekly ward meeting that both the patient and carer can attend. The meetings last for an hour and the focus is on providing information and education to both the patient and their family. The sessions are facilitated by every professional group of the multidisciplinary team on a rotating basis so patients and carers can dip into the particular session that is of relevance to them. Examples of topics covered include psychological and emotional reactions to stroke; what is a stroke?; and the role of the physiotherapist. As well as providing information the sessions also help patients and carers to become aware of the signs of depression so that, hopefully, in the future they will be able more easily to recognise, label and manage the symptoms of depression. This in turn should lead to earlier treatment for depression thereby reducing the impact of the depression on both the patient and the carer.

### Psychosocial interventions for mild depression

The National Institute for Clinical Excellence (2004) produced guidelines for the assessment and treatment of depression. These guidelines are not specifically for patients who have had a stroke but apply to any adult who is suffering from depression. NICE have developed a stepped care model that aims to match the needs of people with depression to the most appropriate service. For example, the first step of the model is the recognition of depression by any professional, whereas the final step on the model relates to those people who are at serious risk of self-harm and who will require input from specialist services and possibly inpatient care. In our service we have used the NICE guidelines to inform our thinking on the treatment of depression in patients who have had a stroke. As Barton (see Chapter 7) discusses, we have developed an Emotional Care Plan to help all members of the team to choose the appropriate assessment tool for measuring mood. Once assessed, staff complete a mood review sheet to monitor the patient's mood and their responses to any interventions. The interventions are chosen from a range of options as recommended by NICE (Table 8.2). Any member of the multidisciplinary team can carry out all the interventions for mild depression. Often staff do not realise that something as straightforward as spending time talking with the patient can be a helpful intervention for mild depression. Patients are aware of all the demands that staff have on their time and are often extremely appreciative of being given a few minutes of time just to

**Table 8.2** Interventions for depression.

| Mild depression | Moderate depression | Severe depression |
| --- | --- | --- |
| Talk with patient | Any from 'Mild depression' | Consider referral to |
| Review goals | *In addition*: | psychiatry |
| Develop discharge plan | Consider antidepressants | *In addition*: |
| Tell Your Story group | Consider psychological | Consider any |
| Agewell group | therapy | intervention for |
| Volunteer input | Discuss with psychologist: | mild to moderate |
| Anxiety management | –problem solving | depression |
| Advice on sleeping | –cognitive behavioural | |
| Discuss options with psychologist | therapy | |

talk rather than for interactions with staff always to be task focused. Because of all the demands on staff time, particularly in hospitals, using volunteer input can be another means of providing activities that will help to improve mood and general well-being. For example, some wards hold regular Agewell Groups where volunteers come onto the wards and provide activities such as arts and crafts, or singing, that provide a distraction from the routine of ward life as well as some meaningful activity. Exercise has been shown to be of benefit for people suffering from depression, and the NICE guidelines recommend that patients with mild depression are advised to follow a structured and supervised programme of exercise for up to three sessions per week (45 minutes to 1 hour) for between 10 and 12 weeks. For the majority of stroke patients this regime would be too demanding but the link between exercise and improved mood is well established, so it is for the team to think of creative ways of adapting this recommendation to suit the needs of the individual patient. Therapy assistants have been very successful in this area and have supported patients to return to gyms with modified exercise programmes or accompanied them swimming.

Helping patients to find some meaningful occupation or activity following their stroke is an important intervention to address symptoms of depression but can be challenging for both the patient and services. Depending on the nature and extent of the disabilities resulting from the stroke the patient may be able to engage in previously enjoyed activities. However, for the majority of patients the challenge is either to engage in former activities in an adapted way or else to try to think of new activities to engage in. The latter often involves a process of grieving or mourning for a past life before feeling emotionally 'free' to expend energy and effort on looking for new interests and activities, as illustrated by Case study 8.1. If someone was working prior to their stroke there is a whole range of issues to be considered in relation to returning to work. For example, are they still able (physically and cognitively) to do the job, can they return to their old job but with changed hours or duties or with adaptations? If they are no longer capable of returning to their former job what type of employment would suit them now? The role of the multidisciplinary team is to help people think through some of the issues in relation to meaningful activities and employment, and on a practical level, practise skills that would be required of them in their meaningful occupation. Finally, the team can also signpost patients to specialist services for further advice and support.

---

**Case Study 8.1 Psychosocial interventions**

Following her stroke, Betty was left with significant expressive aphasia and very limited mobility. She had been in hospital in her home town for many weeks before moving into a Care Home in another city to be near her daughter. Whilst Betty was engaging well in her rehabilitation she was often very distressed and tearful during therapy sessions, which the therapists were becoming concerned about. The psychologist met with Betty and discussed with her the common emotional reactions to stroke and acknowledged all the changes and losses that Betty had experienced as a result of the stroke. Betty admitted that she was concerned that she was losing her mind, but was reassured when the psychologist provided information about grieving and adjusting to those changes and losses. In the course of the session Betty also talked about her activities and interest, and as a result the team were able to facilitate her re-engaging with some of them; for example, she began to go to classical music concerts, and it was arranged for a minister to visit her as she had always been a regular attender at church.

---

## Emotional processing

When people are traumatised by an event, one way of reducing the impact of the trauma is to go over the event to help them emotionally process the information. A 'Tell Your Story' group is one way of emotionally processing the traumatic impact of the stroke. This group is held on the ward and is facilitated by three members of staff and attended by up to six patients. The group meets for about an hour once a week for 3 weeks. The aim of the group is simply to allow people the time and space to tell their story of the stroke and to begin to emotionally process the impact of the stroke and to acknowledge the emotional impact of what has happened to them. It is not about adjusting or coming to terms with the stroke but rather about the very early stages of acknowledging what has happened and beginning to think about the emotional impact. The facilitators use the questions listed below as a guide to structuring the session:

- Where were you when you had your stroke?
- What happened to you?
- When did you realise that you had had a stroke?
- What was it like when you were admitted to hospital?
- What has your stay been like in hospital?

## Goal setting

Setting meaningful, realistic, shared goals is the key to ensuring effective and satisfactory rehabilitation for both the patient and the multidisciplinary team. Given the time constraints (12 weeks) of the Community Rehabilitation Team (CRT) it is vital that patients and their families are provided with information about the service and the professionals who will be visiting their home. In order to facilitate this process a speech and language therapist in our service designed and developed a 'What's Your Goal?' booklet (Haw, 2005). This is an A4 booklet that provides patients and their families with information about the team. A key interest for the author was to ensure that the booklet was accessible to patients with speech and language impairment, who may have particular difficulty reading information or expressing goals. The booklet incorporates picture material. For example, it was felt that the use of the team members' photographs would be of assistance to all patients and carers in helping them to remember and identify the new people who would be visiting them at home. In addition, for patients with speech and language problems, these photographs would provide an immediate way of referring to team members. The written text is simple and presented in both paragraph and bullet point form, so that it looks acceptable but is accessible to as many patients as possible. The main section of the booklet focuses on patients and professionals collaboratively setting individualised goals for the patient. Most of these goals will be achievable within the period that the team is visiting, whilst others will be longer-term goals that the patient will continue to work on, either by themselves or with other services. The booklet is a really helpful tool for engaging patients in rehabilitation and can also help patients maintain their motivation for rehabilitation as patient and therapist can jointly reflect on goals achieved and progress made. Using the booklet with patients who are low in mood has also been useful as bigger goals can be broken down into smaller, more manageable steps. Once a small step has been achieved this can have the effect of positively reinforcing the patient's effort and may provide the patient who has low mood with more impetus and motivation to try to tackle the next step.

## Staff support

In order for members of the multidisciplinary team to feel confident and skilled at carrying out psychological interventions they must have initially received training in this area, which is then backed up by ongoing advice and support. By undertaking psychological interventions we are asking members of the team to engage in a different type of work from their core professional tasks and we should not underestimate the emotional impact that working with emotionally distressed people can have on staff. Staff are not always prepared for the stories they hear, or the depth of emotion that may be expressed by patients. If staff are involved in facilitating groups like Tell Your Story or Stroke Adjustment, colleagues and managers need to be aware that not only is time required to run the group but also adequate time must be made available for planning the group and for debriefing post-group to allow staff the opportunity to reflect on and process what they have heard, as illustrated by Case study 8.2.

---

**Case Study 8.2 Staff support**

Sue was a very experienced therapy assistant who contacted the psychologist following a session with a patient who had expressed suicidal thoughts. In the session with the patient Sue had managed the situation very well and had followed the team's protocol for assessing the risk of suicide (having previously had training on the topic from the psychologist). However, following the session, Sue was very distressed and anxious. By talking it through with the psychologist Sue acknowledged that she had been shocked by the patient's thoughts about not wanting to carry on with life as Sue had felt that rehabilitation was progressing very well and had felt that she had a good relationship with the patient. The psychologist offered to do a joint visit with Sue in order to assess the patient's mood and to discuss whether any further interventions were required (e.g. reviewing progress with goals, antidepressant medication).

---

## Direct interventions

If we refer back to Nichol's model the following interventions are examples of level 3 interventions, which are provided, either entirely or largely, by clinical psychologists in the services we work in.

### Stroke adjustment group

In Sheffield, once people are discharged from hospital they are usually referred to the Community Rehabilitation Team for intensive rehabilitation at home; then, if appropriate, they can be referred on to one of the day rehabilitation units in the city for less intensive but longer-term rehabilitation. As clinical psychologists we became aware that a significant number of our referrals were received either at the point people had recently returned home from hospital or at the point that they were being discharged from rehabilitation services. A frequent reason for referral at these points was that the patient was either 'not coming to terms with the stroke' or was 'anxious about discharge and wishes to continue with rehabilitation despite having reached their potential'. Rather than continue to meet with these patients individually to provide psychological therapy we developed a semi-structured therapeutic group to address the emotional side of coping with a stroke, to try to increase the patients' sense of personal control, and at the same time reduce feelings of helplessness and hopelessness (Barton *et al.*, 2002). The theoretical model on which the group is based is the experience of loss and grieving (shock, denial/disbelief, grief, mourning and depression, anger and hostility, adjustment; Kubler-Ross, 1975). Patients are given the opportunity to share and emotionally process their experiences of the stroke, and to work towards greater psychological acceptance of their disabilities and changed health circumstances.

The groups meet for 2 hours once a week for 6 weeks, and are facilitated by two facilitators and one observer. These roles can either be static or can alternate over the weeks, but a clinical psychologist is always involved in the groups. Other professionals involved have included speech and language therapists, occupational therapists and therapy assistants. Referral criteria are deliberately left quite broad as we feel that most people who have had a stroke would benefit from attending the group. The main exclusion criterion is an inability to understand what is being discussed. A number of groups have included people with an expressive aphasia, who have been able to participate and benefit significantly.

The structure of the group follows a broad planned framework, as outlined in Table 8.3, which allows flexibility to respond to the demands of the group. Each session is based around a theme with group exercises to explore that theme. For example, week 2 focuses on all the changes and losses that people have experienced as a result of their stroke. An individual summary of those changes and losses is written on a flip chart for each person (see example in Table 8.4) and is used again in week 3 when the focus is on the feelings that have been evoked by the changes and losses. Rather than simply ask people spontaneously to discuss their feelings about the stroke we use an exercise called the 'Bag of Feelings'.

**Table 8.3** Stroke Adjustment Group structure.

| Session | Main theme | Content |
|---------|-----------|---------|
| 1 | Emotional processing | The experience of stroke, telling your story, what actually happened, the experience of hospitalisation, associated thoughts and feelings |
| 2 | The experience of loss | Changes and losses associated with stroke, structured exercises |
| 3 | Identification and acknowledgement of feelings | Feelings associated with changes and losses, structured exercises |
| 4 | Understanding thoughts, feelings and behaviour | Thoughts and feelings: introduction to negative thinking and the idea of thinking about your life after stroke. Cognitive-behaviour principles are introduced |
| 5 | Coping | Coping styles and ways of coping are identified and explored. Shared experiences |
| 6 | Summary and evaluation | Individual and group reflections on the group. Gains identified |

**Table 8.4** Example of group exercise for weeks 2 and 3.

| Changes | Losses | Feelings |
|---|---|---|
| Poor balance | Contact with friends | Frustration |
| Spend 90% of time at home | Walking in countryside | Not in control |
| | Loss of role | Old |
| More agitated | Loss of work | Lonely/isolated |
| Become very slow | Hobbies | Angry |
| | The person I was | Frightened |

This exercise involves printed cards with a huge variety of emotions and feelings (both positive and negative) being laid out on the table. Patients are asked to take their time and look through the cards and to pick up any cards that are relevant to them. Finally, the group is asked to share the cards that they have chosen and to talk about them. The feelings are then added to the individual flip charts from week 2. In groups where there have been patients with expressive aphasia we have adapted this task and used more picture-based material, which has worked well. Clinically and anecdotally the Stroke Adjustment Groups appear to be of benefit to a range of stroke patients. Case study 8.3 describes some of these benefits. However, the group is still under development and has yet to be evaluated more rigorously.

---

**Case Study 8.3  Help from a Stroke Adjustment Group**

Six men attended a Stroke Adjustment Group that was held in a Resource Centre. All the men had been affected in different ways by the stroke: mobility problems, enforced retirement, aphasia, having to give up role as a carer and be cared for, changing retirement plans. One of the biggest losses for these men was having to give up driving and the consequent great loss of independence and freedom. The men also talked about the impact of these changes on their relationships with their wives. In some cases the stroke had had a positive impact in that some men reported that it was good to spend more time with their wives. However, most men felt that the stroke had had a negative impact on their relationship and that there was more tension in the household. All the men said that they had lost some confidence since the stroke. One man was particularly honest and open about his feelings and the following are his words: 'At first when I was in hospital I felt very low and cried a lot. At one point I refused to eat. I felt like "a cabbage" and "half a man" and at times I felt like not carrying on with life. I feel cheated that the stroke has disrupted our retirement plans. The fear of having another stroke constantly goes through my mind and at times I have fought going to sleep in case I had another stroke whilst sleeping.'

By the end of the six weeks all the men had moved on and developed ways of coping, e.g. finding solutions to practical problems, using humour to cope, planning holidays. All the men reported that the group had helped them to adjust to the stroke ('the literature that you're given doesn't teach you how to adjust, this group has' 'I've done really well and I must admit that it's due to coming to the group'). One man with aphasia made the following comment at the end of the group: 'One of the things I have found most helpful about the group is that I have had the opportunity to speak. In fact, the first group was the first time since my stroke that I have spoken for so long in front of so many people. I felt good about having spoken so much.'

## Psychological therapy for depression and anxiety

Given the high rates of anxiety symptoms following a stroke it is not surprising that the most common psychological intervention we employ is anxiety management, which includes breathing exercises, physical and mental relaxation, identifying alternative thoughts, and distraction. These approaches can be helpful in tackling most aspects of anxiety, particularly where the anxiety is generalised, and largely related to the person's general rehabilitation and recovery and their plans for the future. Hypnotic or imaginary relaxation techniques can be particularly useful for older people, and people who have had a stroke, where pain might be an issue. The psychologist or occupational therapist can teach the patient basic anxiety management techniques, which can then be reinforced by the rest of the multidisciplinary team. Phobic anxiety (characterised by an unrealistic fear of a particular object, person or situation, which results in avoidant behaviour) is best addressed through the process of systematic desensitisation. In this approach the psychologist, working with the therapy team, helps the patient gradually to make contact with the feared object or situation, through a series of graded steps. The principle here is of approach rather than avoidance of the feared situation. Specific phobias that we have seen following a stroke include: fear of transferring from bed to chair, fear of attempting the stairs, and fear of the place where the stroke happened.

Although there are mixed results regarding the effectiveness of cognitive behaviour therapy (CBT) with stroke patients (Lincoln, Flannaghan, Sutcliffe and Rother, 1997), CBT approaches with older adults have been shown to be effective (Gallagher-Thompson and Thompson, 1996). CBT approaches tend to focus on helping clients to challenge their negative styles of thinking, and to replace these with more adaptive and realistic thinking patterns. This approach can be helpful with stroke patients but needs to take into account any cognitive or communication difficulties and be adapted accordingly. Behaviour therapy is another type of psychological therapy that is known to be helpful for depressed older people. The theory underpinning this is that mood is linked to behaviour, and that by increasing the positive experiences people have, this will lead to an improvement in mood. With stroke patients, building previously enjoyed interests and activities into the day can be extremely helpful.

Most patients who are depressed find it difficult to motivate themselves to engage in activities, and this is where professional involvement is helpful. All members of the multidisciplinary team can help to encourage the patient to participate in activities.

### Psychological therapy for post-traumatic stress disorder (PTSD)

The effects of traumatic experiences, especially in combat situations, have long been recognised. However, more recently, researchers are realising that the potentially life-threatening nature of a stroke can give rise to a traumatic reaction. Recent estimates suggest that 11–15% of people who have had a stroke might experience PTSD. What is probably more common is that many more people may be experiencing some traumatic symptoms, but not necessarily significantly enough to meet diagnostic criteria for PTSD. As with other emotional consequences following a stroke, members of the multidisciplinary team need to have an awareness of the key signs and symptoms of PTSD in order to facilitate a referral to psychology (Box 8.1). Psychological treatment for PTSD involves helping the patient emotionally to process the trauma by focusing on the stroke story in detail and exploring the patient's thoughts and feelings associated with the stroke. The traumatic event of the stroke may cause other emotions related to previous traumatic or stressful experiences to resurface, as described in Case study 8.4. It is worth noting that we have had instances where the carer rather than the patient has been experiencing symptoms of PTSD. This has happened when the carer was present when the patient had the stroke and may have needed to give life-saving interventions until the emergency services arrived.

### Box 8.1   Symptoms of post-traumatic stress disorder (PTSD)

PTSD develops following a stressful event or situation of an exceptionally threatening or catastrophic nature, which is likely to cause pervasive distress in almost anyone. There are three core groups of symptoms:

- *Re-experiencing* the traumatic event in a very vivid and distressing way. This includes flashbacks, nightmares, and distressing and repetitive intrusive images from the event.
- *Avoidance* of reminders about the event—can include people, situations or circumstances that resemble or are associated with the event. For example, one patient changed the route he drove to work, as he did not want to pass the hospital where he had been admitted following his stroke.

- *Hyperarousal*—this includes hypervigilance for threat, exaggerated startle responses, irritability and difficulty concentrating and sleep problems.

---

**Case Study 8.4 Trauma following stroke**

Fiona was a 52-year-old woman who was left with significant visual problems following her stroke but otherwise had physically made a good recovery. However, psychology was asked to see her by CRT because she was extremely anxious in sessions. Psychology ended up working with Fiona for quite some time as there were a number of issues that had arisen as a result of the stroke. Initially, the psychologist helped Fiona and the CRT to set up a graded exposure programme to help Fiona address her anxiety about going outside. Following assessment it was clear that Fiona was experiencing some post-traumatic symptoms, so there was a period of psychological therapy, which focused on Fiona emotionally processing the traumatic event. From this work, it emerged that there were other traumatic events that had occurred earlier in Fiona's life that had resulted in her adopting coping strategies that were not helpful to her in her current situation. The largest piece of work was around issues of adjustment to her life following the stroke and helping her to grieve for the changes and losses and to begin to think about the future and the challenges that lay ahead of her.

---

## Medication

At times medication can be useful and required. Antidepressant medication can be used either alone or in conjunction with psychological therapy where the emotional distress has reached a clinically significant level. For some patients, the depression is so severe that it stops them from engaging in rehabilitation and they require antidepressant medication to lift their mood and to help improve their motivation. Depending on which part of the service the patient is in when their depression is recognised and assessed will determine which health professional will be prescribing the medication, for example hospital consultant or GP. In order to provide some guidance to doctors we have a number of protocols in place within the city that offer specific advice on which antidepressants are most effective in managing post-stroke depression and emotionalism. The protocols also outline when a referral to specialist mental health services should be made; i.e. following failure to respond to two antidepressants or where there is severe depression or serious suicidal intent.

## Cognitive problems following stroke

Whilst the focus of this chapter has been on psychological approaches to working with the emotional consequences of stroke, the cognitive changes that can result from a stroke have a huge impact on both the patient and their families. In the early days following a stroke, the majority of patients experience some cognitive problems (British Psychological Society, 2002). These typically include:

1. *Confusion and disorientation*. Patients are often unaware of the time, where they are, or what has happened to them.
2. *Memory problems*. These might include remembering important information about themselves and their families, remembering new information, or remembering recent events that have happened.
3. *Concentration*. Problems often manifest during therapy sessions, or when patients are attempting to read a book, or watch a television programme.
4. *Perceptual problems*. These might include problems with the detection of shapes in space, or indeed of themselves in space.
5. *Executive functioning*. Problems are often associated with reasoning and planning, and with initiation and regulation of behaviour.
6. *Attention*. Problems tend to be characterised in terms of dividing, switching, selecting or sustaining attention.

Many of these cognitive problems resolve over time, but approximately 35% of people who survive a stroke will be left with longer-term cognitive impairment (Tatemichi *et al.*, 1994). The RCP's Guidelines recommend that all patients should be screened for the presence of cognitive impairments as soon as is practicable. Routine assessment of cognitive functioning is usually undertaken with a screening instrument, and followed up with in-depth specialist assessments if problems are detected. Screening measures used in our service include the Mini-Mental State Examination (Folstein and McHugh, 1975) and the Middlesex Elderly Assessment of Mental State (Golding, 1989). In selecting more in-depth assessments, it is important first to define the question to be answered, and to think about what information may actually be helpful. Where the patient has communication impairment, the use of standardised measures may not be appropriate, and assessment may need to be undertaken through observation. On the basis of results, various strategies might be suggested by the psychologist or occupational therapist to aid rehabilitation. Box 8.2 provides some examples.

### Box 8.2   Strategies for working with cognitive impairment

**Problems with executive functioning**
- General principle is to provide structure
- Plan and talk through a task prior to activity

- Continually prompt and guide through a task
- Encourage self-reflection and monitoring of behaviour

**Memory problems**
- Encourage patients to use external memory aids, e.g. diaries, electronic organisers, dictaphones
- Simplify information and provide written instructions
- Divide information into small chunks
- Use errorless learning techniques

**Attention and concentration problems**
- Minimise unnecessary distractions
- Focus on one thing at a time
- Provide warning and preparation that the patient needs to switch their attention to a new task

In some cases, cognitive assessments may be requested in order to answer very specific questions, such as 'is the person fit to return to driving?' In our service we began to recognise that an increasing number of patients were entering rehabilitation with a desire to return to driving as their main therapy goal. This raised a number of issues for us, including: which cognitive assessments to use, how to ensure information regarding legal requirements and DVLA (Driver and Vehicle Licensing Agency) regulations was provided consistently across the care pathway, and how to improve communication between primary and secondary care. A multidisciplinary working party has taken on this large project and has started to address some of the complex issues surrounding this area. So far, we have produced an information leaflet for professionals outlining the legal obligations regarding duty of care to patients and actions to be taken. Information leaflets have also been produced for patients explaining how driving may be affected after a stroke and also what the assessment process involves. A comprehensive cognitive assessment battery has been compiled based upon both the literature and practicalities, such as, ensuring that the assessments chosen could be administered by occupational therapists. Other strands to the project have included on-road assessments and standardising the feedback process to primary care. This work is ongoing and the latest phase is for us to begin to consider how these assessments may be adapted for patients with communication impairment.

## Conclusions

A stroke is a traumatic life-threatening and life-changing event that can leave people with significant emotional, cognitive, physical, behavioural and social difficulties that encompass all areas of a person's life and functioning. Psychological and emotional care must begin as soon as the individual experiencing the stroke, and their family, make contact with healthcare services. The psychological and emotional care can either be provided via direct means, such as psychological therapy, or, as is hopefully more often the case, indirectly, through every communication and interaction that the patient and their family have with professionals on their recovery journey. For psychological approaches to be successful they need to be adopted by all members of the multidisciplinary team and to be creative in adapting to the needs of individual patients. One of the challenges facing services is how to provide emotional care in the longer term for those patients who may not experience the full psychological impact of the stroke until long after they have been discharged from physical rehabilitation services.

## References

Barton J, Miller A, Chanter J. Emotional adjustment to stroke: a group therapeutic approach. Nursing Times 2002;98:33–35.

British Psychological Society. Psychological Services for Stroke Survivors and their Families. Briefing paper 19. Leicester: British Psychological Society, 2002.

Folstein S, McHugh P. Mini-Mental State: A practical method for grading the cognitive state of patients for the clinician. J Psychiatr Res 1975;12:189–198.

Gallagher-Thompson D, Thompson L. Applying cognitive behavioural therapy to the psychological problems of later life. In: Zarit SH, Knight BG (eds) A Guide to Psychotherapy and Ageing. Washington, DC: American Psychological Association, 1996.

Golding E. Middlesex Elderly Assessment of Mental State. London: Thames Valley Test Company, 1989.

Haw C. 'Do you have a master plan?' Speech and Language Therapy in Practice. Laurencekirk: Avril Nicoll, 2005.

Kubler-Ross E. Death: The Final Stage of Growth. New York: Prentice Hall, 1975.

Lincoln N, Flannaghan T, Sutcliffe L, Rother L. Evaluation of cognitive behavioural treatment for depression after stroke: a pilot study. Clin Rehabil 1997;11:114–122.

Moos RH, Tsu VD. The crisis of physical illness. In: Moos RH (ed.) Coping with Physical Illness. New York: Plenum, 1977.

National Institute for Clinical Excellence. The Treatment of Depression in Adults. London: NICE, 2004.

Nichols K. Psychological care for ill and injured people: a clinical guide. Maidenhead: Open University Press, 2003.

Nichols K. Why is psychology still failing the average patient? Psychologist 2005;18:26–27.

Royal College of Physicians. National Clinical Guidelines for Stroke, 2nd edn. London: Royal College of Physicians, 2004.

Stroke Association. 'Nobody Told Me'. Briefing paper. London: Stroke Association, 2006.

Tatemichi TK, Desmond DW, Stern Y, Palik M, Sano M, Bagella E. Cognitive impairments after stroke: frequency, patterns, and relationships to functional abilities. J Neurol Neuorsurg Psych 1994;57:202–207.

# CHAPTER 9

# Group Therapy — An Interprofessional Approach

## Diane Brown and Mairi Knox

This chapter is a reflection of the experiences of a multidisciplinary team (MDT) in their development and running of a group for stroke patients. The group took place on an acute stroke rehabilitation unit. It was intended to promote and support well-being and understanding of the changes clients may have been experiencing following their stroke. This chapter will explore the development, running and effects of the group on both the staff on the unit and the clients who participated in it. It is hoped that the chapter proves a useful account of the benefits and difficulties in running such a group and will be of practical use to anyone wishing to replicate it.

## Development of the group

### Derivation of the group

Stroke is the single most common cause of severe disability within the UK. Every year over 130 000 people in the UK have a stroke, that is one person every 5 minutes. Most people affected are over 65, but anyone can have a stroke. Stroke is usually a sudden and often devastating event for those it affects. More than 250 000 people live with disabilities caused by stroke. Despite the prevalence of stroke it remains a condition that is difficult to understand due to the range and diversity of symptoms that individuals experience. It is often said that no two strokes are the same (Stroke Association, 2007). It is the experience of the authors that patients' and families' understanding of stroke tend to be limited to the more obvious physical disabilities. Communicative, cognitive and psychosocial implications, and their impact on self-esteem, are less overt and as a result are not as widely recognised. This is reflected in service provision, where assistance with promoting physical recovery and resuming activities of daily living tends to be the focus of rehabilitation. However, the second edition of the Royal College of Physicians' Guidelines for stroke (Royal College of Physicians, 2004) has increased focus on these areas; examples of their recommendations (under section 4, 'Rehabilitation') include: 'Patients' psychological and social needs should be assessed' (p. 53); 'All patients should be screened for the presence of cognitive impairment as soon as is practicable. The nature of the impairment should be determined, and its impact on activity and participation should be explained to patients, careers and staff' (p. 56); 'If the patient has aphasia the staff and relatives should be informed and trained by the speech and language therapists about communication techniques appropriate to the communication disability' (p. 60).

The context for the group is a town in the north of England with a population of 218 100 spread over an area of 127 square miles. It has strong contrasts between countryside and urban industrial areas. It includes the main town and other smaller towns and former mining villages. The area is not culturally diverse in that 98% of its population are white British.

Within the area covered by the Primary Care Trust there are an average of 500 strokes a year (local figures collated and provided by stroke nurse consultant). The stroke rehabilitation unit is located in a small (three wards) subacute rehabilitation hospital. At the time of the group development the unit consisted of 12 adult patients both male and female. The majority of patients were admitted onto the unit approximately 8–10 days following their stroke, from the local District General Hospital. Patients' length of stay on the unit varied but was usually no longer than 10–12 weeks. Of the patients on the unit 60–70% had communication and or cognitive impairment, whilst most had mobility impairments of varying degrees.

The group evolved as a result of MDT discussions within formal (team meetings, supervision, goal setting) and informal (session feedback, problem-solving, morning handover) settings. The team or MDT described within this chapter consisted of physiotherapists (two full-time), speech and language therapists (one full-time equivalent), occupational therapists (two full-time), dietician (3½ days a week), clinical psychologist (1 day a week), generic therapy assistant (one full-time), nursing staff and rehabilitation assistants. All professionals were located within the same working environment, which offered maximum opportunity for sharing experiences and ideas. Many members of the team were highly experienced within their profession and within the clinical area of stroke rehabilitation. Team discussions highlighted a significant gap in the service we were providing, despite offering patients intensive therapeutic support at an impairment level. The gap was identified as an unmet need to provide regular emotional support and opportunity to deal with the early impact of stroke. Some clients found it difficult to focus on therapy tasks if their priorities were to understand the changes to their lives and to grieve over the loss of their previously held roles. Recurrent themes they raised included: a reluctance to worry family/careers, pain, sleep, toileting, loss of self-esteem, future roles, not being understood, eating and relationships. To address this, it was found that clients regularly sought reassurance and information whenever, in a quiet and secure environment with a professional. Others were reluctant to participate in therapy or ward activities, suggesting 'It will be alright when I get home'.

This impacted on the service in two ways:

1. Professionals found they were often spending up to half of planned therapeutic sessions either listening to and dealing with clients' emotional responses to the stroke, or answering questions and imparting information. Although the team acknowledged the value of this intervention it did not leave sufficient time to make optimum progress with more impairment-based therapy.
2. Concerns arose that all staff were dealing with similar client issues but possibly in unstructured and unplanned ways, which varied depending on the clients' symptoms (particularly cognitive and communication deficits) and the professionals' experience of them. This may have resulted in issues not being addressed optimally and thus leaving the client feeling isolated and frustrated.

Taking the above observations into account, it was agreed that both the clients and the service would benefit from the development of a group to address the issues highlighted in our team discussions. The MDT undertook some research within the local area and through journal articles to identify similar groups that may already have been developed. Although our research was not extensive, we found that groups already in existence were running with clients at a later stage of their recovery, i.e. in the community, or they were facilitated uniprofessionally (Barton, Miller and Chanter, 2002; Van der Gaag et al., 2005). This suggested to us that a new approach would be to develop a group that could include any client and was facilitated by a multidisciplinary team instead of one professional.

The following section highlights the questions we felt needed justifying prior to allocating time and resources to development of such a group.

## Why a group?

All clients, unless medically unfit, received regular one-to-one therapy from individual professions during their stay on the unit. However, one-to-one work does not capitalise upon the substantial contribution that other clients can make to the recovery of each other by providing mutual emotional support, a sounding board, a feeling of being part of a group and confronting the same challenge. Bray and Todd (2006) concur with this view suggesting 'The client is not confined to interactions with the clinician and any other attendant person concentrating solely on his or her own case, but participants in therapy related to the needs, concerns and behaviours of other clients too'.

The group would give clients an opportunity to compare themselves with others in a similar position and reduce feelings of isolation. Individuals with a similar diagnosis could use group sessions to solve common issues that directly affected their quality of life. The group could also provide them with a sense of value in offering support to others rather than being the constant recipient of help (Markus and Nurius, 1986; Luterman, 1996; Kurtz, 1997).

Communication-impaired/cognitively impaired clients were often reluctant to speak on the unit, and the group could provide a safe place in which to desensitise them to these issues and allow them to practice developing skills and build confidence. A group environment promotes group interaction among members, which should foster skills such as turn taking, attention and initiation, and incorporate more natural interactions. Peer modelling within the group and an opportunity to practice strategies provided in one-to-one therapy may increase the likelihood of generalising these skills to home and community environments.

Traditional relationships between therapist and client often involve the client being the 'recipient' and the therapists a 'provider'. This can result in a more 'passive' client who feels less in control of the rehabilitation process, which reduces their participation in it. The group would provide clients with an opportunity to move into an arena of being 'active' participants where they are able to direct or lead the themes discussed. This may offer clients a bridge from a sense of passivity and dependency on professionals to a sense of being more in control of their rehabilitation. In turn this should allow them to participate more confidently and appropriately in goal-setting sessions by offering the beginnings of some individual control. It was hoped that the group would make an early move towards creating a less dependent practitioner–client relationship. This would also be of benefit as clients progressed through to discharge from therapeutic intervention. Our group further reduced the risk of dependency on therapists by being open (as opposed to a closed group where members remain constant throughout its duration), and having rotating facilitators, an issue that is addressed further in the following section.

The group aimed to promote emotional recovery from a stroke as a process of clients learning both about themselves and about the support that is available to assist them. It was hoped that the benefits of attending a group would have a positive impact on the clients' self-esteem, which could be measured pre- and post-group attendance.

### Why a multidisciplinary team?

It was felt that it was a priority to utilise the skills of the multidisciplinary team in order to develop and run the group. The benefits of this were:

- A broad range of skills were on hand, allowing for all possible deficits to be addressed and therefore the clients' needs to be considered more holistically.

- Staff would gain a knowledge and understanding of each other's skills rarely afforded in normal practice of case load management. This would allow individual clinicians to have a greater skill base from which to draw when working as an individual practitioner.
- The time spent preparing for and running the group was shared between professions. Logistically this meant that no one profession was depleted to an extent that usual one-to-one therapy could not continue alongside the group.
- Working as a team makes devising and measuring the group more objective (i.e. provides inter-rater reliability).

In developing the group we were aware that different facilitators would bring varying skills and experiences. We felt that it was important to maintain continuity, which was promoted by clear group aims, topic structure and an observer being present through one group rotation who would be a facilitator within the next group. To aid levels of continuity within the group, junior members of staff worked alongside a more experienced staff member.

## Why all deficits?

In our experience previous groups run on the unit tended to be unidisciplinary and address a specific issue, for example upper limb, memory, relaxation, or anxiety management. This limited opportunities for talking about other concerns. In addition, groups for specific issues often excluded clients with communication or cognitive deficits. We were therefore keen to ensure that all clients had an equal opportunity to attend and participate in the group. The issues to be addressed (well-being) were of equal relevance to all clients regardless of their deficits and so the group allowed equal access.

This group is an early opportunity within a safe environment to explore and challenge with other clients who are also dealing with life adjustments but not all in exactly the same way. Bray and Todd (2006) suggest that 'as long as each member can achieve personal objectives within the group experience, and there are also some mutually acceptable objectives, members need not have common features on terms of such things as background and type and severity of communication disorder' (p. 34).

## Aims of the group

The aims of the group evolved naturally as the need for the group was acknowledged and developed. A written summary of the aims is provided in Box 9.1, first as we developed it, and below in the form that it was presented to the group.

## Box 9.1 Development and final summary of aims of the group

**Purpose, aims and objectives of the group**

The purpose of the group was to improve clients' self-esteem, provide a sense of self-control and an awareness of potential for further recovery.

This was to be achieved through the following aims and objectives:

*Aim 1*

To facilitate discussion around specific stroke-related topics encompassing emotional, physiological, social, personal and future needs of the client.

*Objectives:*

- The group will be facilitated by two members (and observed/supported by one other) of the multidisciplinary team.
- Team members will facilitate the group for a period of 5 weeks at which time the two lead facilitators will rotate.

*Aim 2*

To provide a regular forum in which clients can obtain support and information from professionals and other members of the group.

*Objectives:*

- The group will meet for 90 minutes every week.
- An appropriate environment will be utilised.
- Resources offering information relevant to the needs and understanding of clients will be produced and provided.

*Aim 3*

Greater social contact to reduce the feeling of isolation that clients can experience following a stroke.

*Objective:*

- All patients on the stroke Rehabilitation Unit will be invited to attend the group.

*Aim 4*

To allow the clients to anticipate and prepare for their future rather than to focus solely on the 'here and now'.

To give clients a sense of a 'stroke journey' and allow them to set their own goals for future recovery.

*Objectives:*
- Group discussion will be structured around the idea of clients being on a 'stroke journey'. This will be facilitated by the use of drawings and diagrams showing an individual's progress through different stages of recovery, i.e. acute stages, rehabilitation, and discharge from hospital and onto achieving an optimal quality of life.

**Aims of the group**
1. WE WILL TALK ABOUT STROKE, OURSELVES AND HOW WE FEEL
2. WE WILL MEET EVERY WEDNESDAY MORNING
3. WE WILL GIVE YOU FACTS ABOUT YOUR STROKE
4. WE WILL ALL HELP EACH OTHER IF WE CAN
5. WE WILL PLAN FOR LEAVING HOSPITAL

## Structure of the group

The practicalities of the group needed addressing to ensure that the group could run competently each week and for the 5-week rotation period. We felt that the following questions needed to be answered.

### How would it be staffed?

Two facilitators from different professions would run the group for a 5-week period and then hand over to two new facilitators. This is what staffing would allow for, and two different professions would provide a more holistic approach, as discussed previously. The facilitators were all qualified professionals including speech and language therapists, occupational therapists, physiotherapists and a dietician. It would be organised at least 10 weeks in advance in our diaries to ensure minimal need for cancellation of the group. In the running of the group a facilitator from the next rotation also participated, both to observe the current rotation to allow continuity of group skills and to give one-to-one support to those clients who needed greater assistance in contributing. Although nursing staff contributed to the development of the group they were unable to facilitate due to shift patterns preventing regular weekly time slots.

### Who would attend?

Everyone who attended had had a stroke (diagnosed by CT scan or medical consultants' diagnosis) and was currently resident on the Stroke Rehabilitation Unit. The only exclusion from attending the group was being medically unfit. Clients who did not overtly display an emotional reaction to the affects of their stroke were actively encouraged to attend the group as clients displaying a less emotive response were still adjusting to the stroke, albeit in a more covert manner. The experience of the team showed that in the early stages clients respond to and cope with the effects of their stroke in various ways, from denial of the event to uncontrolled tearfulness. Indeed, clients who appeared to seek less emotional support were often in greater need for an avenue in which to express their internal thoughts, feelings and concerns.

## How many could attend?

On average eight to ten clients were medically fit enough to attend the group, and this was accepted as a suitable number for the staffing already allocated.

## Where and when would the group be held?

Ideally staff would have liked the group to have been held in an environment outside the unit to provide clients with a sense of separation from their 'hospital role'. In organising the group this was not achievable on a consistent basis, so the next best option was to use the quietest room available within the Stroke Rehabilitation Unit. Other considerations when choosing the venue were:

- size of room
- availability of tables
- privacy
- comfortable chairs
- easy access to refreshments and toilets.

The group ran from 10:30 am to 12:00 noon, a time of day that was best in terms of clients' alertness and energy levels. This was also an optimal time in that visiting on the unit was in the afternoon. Allocating a regular time slot allowed staff on the Stroke Rehabilitation Unit to allocate other tasks to their day, while the majority of the clients were absent.

## Resources

In developing a group that allowed all clients equal access we identified the difficulty in enabling those clients with communication and cognitive impairments to participate. With this in mind we strove to design and resource the group accordingly. Visual, symbolic and pictorial objects in the form of black-and-white line drawings or photographs, and the use of large print 'keywords', were all developed and trialled with communication- and cognitively impaired clients in one-to-one therapy sessions prior to their use within the group. Analogue Likert scales were used to rate clients' responses during different activities and discussions during the groups (Figure 9.1). Simplified written handouts were provided

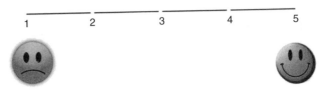

**Figure 9.1** Example of Likert scales used within the group.

as a reference to the content of each group and as a tool to aid discussion with the clients' families; these were especially of use to clients with memory impairments. Silent resources took the form of facilitators modifying communication to maximize clients' understanding of the information presented and the use of gesture based on the Makaton system. Whilst these skills were easier for those professionals developing the group (occupational therapist and speech and language therapist) these were newly acquired skills for other professionals who became facilitators. These skills were reported as useful in their one-to-one therapy sessions. Other resources that were found to be helpful included whiteboards, chunky marker pens and pen aids.

A large picture showing a winding road along which a client would travel during their recovery from a stroke was adapted from a line drawing featured in a brochure *Communication Impairments Following Stroke* from the Stroke Association (brochure now out of print). Along the road were displayed separate pictures representing people, places and activities that clients may encounter during their journey. For example, at the beginning of the roadway was a representation of the client at 'home' before the stroke, moving along to a picture of the acute hospital and the client in bed.

### Plans for measuring the group

It was of prime importance, when developing the group, to establish a method of measuring its outcomes. The method chosen would have to be accessible to all clients and provide enough detail to capture more discrete changes. The reasons for carrying out this evaluation were to:

- assess the usefulness of the group to clients;
- make improvements for future groups;
- measure changes in a client's emotional state;
- provide evidence to support the future running of the group.

This was evaluated using the following tools:

- Visual Analogue Self-Esteem Scale (Brumfitt and Sheeran, 1999);
- Non-Sexist Blob Tree (Wilson, 1988) (now obtainable: Wilson and Long, 2008);
- simple questionnaire (developed by staff on the unit).

These tools were completed by the two facilitators who would be responsible for running that group rotation. The same facilitator would complete both the post- and pre-group measure in an individual session during the two or three days prior to the initial session or after the final session. Any changes noticed in the measure were highlighted and discussed with the client in the post-group session.

Standardised assessments and checklists such as the Hospital Anxiety and Depression Scale (Zigmond and Snaith, 1983), with the exception of the VASES, were not used as they were found to be inappropriate for some clients due to their reliance on the use of more complex language. It was acknowledged that this would limit the measuring of outcome; however, we felt that capturing the experience of clients normally excluded from such data was of more value than a more complete measure of fewer clients.

## Running the group

This section will cover a description of the group agreement and session plans, highlighting themes and topics included each week. It will give examples of specific resources used.

### Group agreement

As the title suggests, the group agreement comprised a set of guidelines agreed upon by participants and facilitators to support the cohesion of the group. They were presented and discussed at the beginning of each group; a need for change was never identified. When presenting the agreement (Box 9.2) it was occasionally necessary to clarify individual points.

### Box 9.2   Group agreement

- EVERYONE MUST HAVE A CHANCE TO SPEAK
- LISTEN TO OTHERS WHEN THEY ARE SPEAKING
- WHAT IS SAID IN THE GROUP IS PRIVATE
- HELP EACH OTHER TO SAY WHAT WE MEAN
- IF IT IS HARD TO TALK IT IS OK JUST TO LISTEN
- IT IS OK TO LEAVE THE GROUP IF YOU NEED TO

### Session plans

All the sessions followed a similar format. At the start of the session, after reviewing group guidelines, the facilitator introduced the topic of the week using pictures, or keywords. Each topic was then related to a pictorial representation of the 'stroke journey', identifying the relevance of issues to pre-, present and post-stroke (Box 9.3). For example, topics discussed in Week 4 'Relationships' would first be talked about from the perspective of an individual prior to their stroke. This would then move on to how clients felt this had changed since they were in hospital, with an increased possibility of them feeling more reliant on family and friends. Discussion would end with looking forwards and planning for the future in maintaining current relationships and forging new ones.

## Box 9.3 'Living with Stroke Group' programme

### Session 1: Information about stroke
- introduce Stroke Journey;
- clarify clients' current understanding of stroke;
- education around stroke, including aetiology, relating symptoms to area and severity of lesion;
- discuss the differing presenting symptoms of the group;
- benefits of rehabilitation;
- identifying possible lifestyle changes to avoid the recurrence of stroke.

### Session 2: Health issues
- discuss basic health needs, e.g. pain, sleep, eating, toileting, breathing, mobility;
- relate above to 'Stroke Journey' to acknowledge any changes from pre- to post-stroke;
- discuss current health issues, e.g. medication, diet, blood pressure checks;
- discuss future health needs, follow-up clinic, GP involvement, further rehabilitation.

### Session 3: Impairments in common
- clients telling their story;
- sharing common experiences;
- supporting each other;
- emotional impact of stroke, coping with change;
- discuss possible support now and in the future (relate to Stroke Journey).

### Session 4: Relationships
- share previously held roles and relationships (work, home, friends);
- current support networks;
- coping with changes in own role;
- discuss sustaining relationships in the future.

**Session 5: Interests and hobbies**
- discussing previous interests;
- ideas to incorporate interests and hobbies into rehabilitation, e.g. options of other groups, gardening, crosswords, music, art;
- finding new ways of enjoying ourselves (use 'Stroke Journey');
- options for support in the future to maintain leisure and hobbies (e.g. Stroke Group, Speakability Group, supported holidays, disabled sports).

### Facilitator's role

During sessions the facilitator's role was:

- to present the topics ensuring a common understanding;
- to encourage shared discussion;
- to ensure equal participation of clients where possible;
- to ensure a general adherence to themes discussed;
- to assist the group in overcoming difficulties, e.g. communication, emotions, over-talkers, reluctance to join in;
- to draw each session to a close.

Short summarising notes (group evaluation summary) were completed by group facilitators at the end of each session to highlight:

- beneficial content
- problem areas
- possible changes to future groups.

## Case Studies

The following case studies attempt to capture the backgrounds, changes due to stroke and individual group involvement of three participants. In Case studies 9.1–9.3 we have tried to offer examples of the differing issues that participants were dealing with, and our experiences of adjusting the group to meet their individual needs.

### Case Study 9.1 Low confidence after the stroke

Mrs X, a 33-year-old married woman and mother of a 12-year-old son and 3-month-old daughter, had a left hemisphere stroke. She presented with moderate to severe comprehension and expressive language impairments. Mrs X had a right-sided weakness affecting both her upper and lower limbs. On admission to the unit she was unable to mobilise; however, upon discharge she could walk short distances unaided. Impaired insight resulted in passivity and difficulties engaging in therapy and goal setting. She was reluctant to communicate with other people on the unit and often appeared embarrassed if they initiated conversation with her. She even appeared self-conscious around her own family, as she refused to practise language activities with them. As a result she actively avoided interaction with staff and other clients, keeping to her room as much as possible.

Mrs X's introduction to the group required extra time and adapted explanations so she could make a more informed decision regarding attendance. Completing the VASES prior to the group allowed an opportunity to discuss the emotions it elicited with Mrs X and to confirm that these topics would be addressed further within the group. She eventually agreed to attend a session with the proviso that she could leave should she feel uncomfortable. We acknowledged her reticence to attend but encouraged her to do so, hoping that this could ultimately be of benefit to her.

During her first session, Mrs X was quiet, listening and watching others during discussion. There were others in the group with communication difficulties, which she became aware of, and she did not seem uncomfortable with the content or situation. Staff on the unit noticed that during the week following the group she interacted more with certain members of staff on the unit.

Mrs X agreed more willingly to attend a second session, which was about lifestyles and hobbies. She seemed keen to share ideas, and with the support of the staff and other group members she selected symbols and words to identify hobbies she enjoyed. Subsequent to this session staff again noticed a change in her behaviour. There was a perceived increase in motivation during therapy sessions and she started to communicate therapy goals and make choices of other activities on the unit. Eventually Mrs X became a more confident member of the group, occasionally taking a mentoring role with other clients, particularly those with communication difficulties. Through the period that she attended the group there was a marked improvement in her insight of her own situation. She engaged in setting appropriate goals for her rehabilitation, such as becoming more independent in caring for her new baby. Her confidence and inclination to communicate (by whatever means possible) increased, enabling her to be an active participant in her rehabilitation.

Pre-group VASES score = 32
Post-group VASES score = 38

Before the group Mrs X tended to select the score in the middle range of options on the scale; this may have been due to her lack of understanding, reduced insight or denial of the impact of the stroke. The VASES score after the group would suggest an increased understanding of her difficulties, for example as she was recognising that she could not always be *understood*, and was sometimes *mixed up*. This, alongside her changed behaviour, indicated a more active approach to rehabilitation.

---

### Case Study 9.2 Limited self-awareness after the stroke

Mrs B was a 65-year-old widow who had lived alone and independently prior to her stroke. She had two adult sons who were supportive of her situation. Her stroke had left her with severe expressive language impairments in that her expression consisted mainly of jargon; she also had moderate receptive impairments. She had difficulty with divided attention, prospective memory impairments and some evidence of dyspraxia. Although able to walk she was unsteady on her feet and required close supervision. Within the ward environment she was always observed to be chatting with other clients and relatives, watching television and reading books despite her inability to engage in these activities at the same level prior to her stroke. Mrs B was an enthusiastic active participant within the group from the first session.

She was prone to give long monologues, which were difficult to understand, and rarely used resources that would have aided her communication. She struggled to self monitor and so had a poor awareness of the impact of her limited communication on other group members. At the initial group, facilitators modelled how to use communication tools, such as non-verbal communication techniques, and how to check that people understood her message. In subsequent groups other group members became skilled at using these techniques to support Mrs B to have a more interactive communication style. It seemed less confrontational to address these issues within a supportive group setting rather than continually working on conversations that were contrived during specific speech therapy sessions. These skills were observed to be generalised into other interactions taking place outside the group, such as at the dinner table. Mrs B had a lot of family members, who tended to visit together; this had previously been difficult for her to cope with, and had left her and her family feeling frustrated (as identified during VASES assessment and through discussion with family during carers' group). The skills she learned during group conversation increased her awareness of her own communication and allowed her to adapt it more effectively, thereby reducing her frustration.

On readministering the VASES after the group, Mrs B scored herself as less frustrated and angry.

Pre-group VASES score = 44
Post-group VASES score = 39

Prior to the group Mrs B scored herself as having no impairments within any area other than regularly feeling frustrated and angry. Subsequent to the group her scores in other domains changed, which may be due to some acknowledgement of her difficulties as a result of the stroke. However, her frustration and anger were scored as less frequent. Her family attending a relatives' support group reported to staff that Mrs B appeared 'more settled' following her attendance of the group over a period of 5 weeks.

## Case Study 9.3 Difficulty in showing feelings after the stroke

Mr Y was a 54-year-old man who was divorced; however, his ex-wife was extremely supportive during his rehabilitation. He had been active and working full time prior to the stroke, but his ex-wife reported that his social life was limited to close family and he was living in a bed-sit. Mr Y had a right hemisphere stroke that left him with moderate left-sided neglect, poor mobility and reduced initiation in daily activities including self-care and feeding. His communicative interactions and emotional response to the devastating affects of his stroke were negligible; for example, his only initiation during the day was to ask staff if he could go outside for a cigarette. He agreed to attend the group and evaluated himself as having low self-esteem during completion of the VASES. He participated in five group sessions, in which he made minimal contribution, although during the group discussing social relationships and emotions he did become tearful. When asked, he chose not to divulge any information about what may have triggered this response; however, he wished to remain in the group and became tearful on further occasions as other members also expressed their sadness. On further discussion following this group he requested a session with the clinical psychologist, something he had previously refused.

Although Mr Y never fully engaged in conversations within the group, the setting did allow him to acknowledge feelings and seek help for this. On readministration of the VASES following the group, his score seemed to indicate an improvement in his overall self-esteem; this was also reflected in his clinical psychology sessions.

Pre-group VASES score = 26
Post-group VASES score = 32

## Effects of the group

In planning and running the group, provision was not made to evaluate it in a standardised way; indeed, it would almost be impossible ethically to eliminate all factors influencing a client's progress and well-being (other than the group) in order for this to be achieved. For example, every client attending the group had varied influencing medical factors, was also receiving one-to-one therapy, was participating in other group work, and had differing levels of family/career support.

### Structured group evaluation

The results gathered from clients (either when a client had attended all five sessions or on discharge) through completion of the VASES, Non-Sexist Blob Tree (Wilson, 1988) and the simple questionnaire suggested that the group was effective in achieving its overall aims.

### VASES

The majority of clients demonstrated a change in their score from pre- to post-group attendance. These scores need to be considered on an individual basis as a change in score either up or down may reflect a positive change. For example, a client starting with a very high score may then show a decrease in their score following the group. At first sight this may seem to show a negative impact of the group, but in fact may highlight an individual who previously had impairments in accepting their difficulties. However, the majority of clients showed a moderate increase in their score. A common theme was noted in that clients showed a greater increase in the following domains after attending group sessions:

- Confidence
- Cheerfulness
- Optimism
- Frustration

**Non-sexist blob tree**

This non-verbal pictorial activity was completed by clients to establish their view of themselves within the Stroke Journey. It formed a useful tool for discussion and reflection prior to completing the initial pre-group VASES. At the beginning of the groups, most clients depicted themselves at the very bottom of the tree moving up with support from others; some clients identified themselves as alone or isolated. Occasionally clients added words to qualify their choice; for example, one client placed himself on a ledge on the side of the tree and wrote 'If not careful will drop off edge'. After completing attendance of the group the Non-Sexist Blob Tree was revisited. Clients generally placed themselves higher up the tree, in a more supported position (often with others) and selected the images with happier faces. A comment from one client when completing this was 'I know I'll get there with help'.

**Living with stroke group questionnaire**

This questionnaire was developed to support clients in giving individual feedback about their experience of the group. The format of the questionnaire was structured to help those with communication impairment, i.e. a short statement followed by a yes or no response. Comments were encouraged if the client was able to expand upon feedback; for example: 'We tried to provide information about stroke. Was this easy to follow? Have some of your concerns or worries been covered in the group?' Most clients, on completing this, limited their responses to 'Yes' or 'No'. In general clients were satisfied with the topics and level of information, and indicated they felt more supported and less worried after attending the group. We also received some useful comments such as:

'If we are very worried about something we can ask for help from others'
'I know more about my stroke'
'Can I get some help with my benefits?'

**Informal evaluation of the group**

Views and opinions within this section were gathered from feedback from observers of the group, family members and carers, mostly while attending the careers' group (this was a weekly group held in the evening, facilitated by the stroke nurse consultant/stroke nurse co-ordinator to support families/carers, and other team members working on the unit). The facilitator's contribution was based on experiences of running the groups and through documentation from the group evaluation summary sheets (Box 9.4).

## Box 9.4  Summary of the positive aspects of the group gathered from carers' and staff comments

- Staff reported less time spent dealing with emotional and educational aspects of stroke during individual rehabilitation sessions, therefore maximising time spent on actual therapy.
- Staff reported that clients appeared to be more aware of reasons and need for individual therapy, and so more motivated to attend.
- Staff observed improved participation in client-led goal setting.
- Clients noted to be more overt in acknowledging the need for support now and in anticipating their discharge (usually home) particularly observed during discharge planning meeting.
- Staff reported fewer demands on time spent resolving client and carer issues.
- Clients with communication and cognitive impairments were reported to be less reticent in trying strategies to interact outside the group or individual treatment sessions.
- Staff within follow-on services (seeing patients within the community) reported patients mentioning participation in the group and friendships made. Participants from the group were reported to be more at ease within community groups.
- Carers reported (either in a one-to-one or within carers' group) that family members appeared less anxious and more interactive.

### Benefits and difficulties of the group

Some of the benefits and difficulties experienced in the running of the group were expected. Many benefits demonstrated an achievement of our aims, others were less expected but no less valuable. Running a group is never going to be problem free, particularly in view of the range of deficits, personalities and life experiences that people bring to it. No amount of planning can avoid hitches; as a result, difficulties were not necessarily viewed in a negative way but as part of a learning experience and used to improve future groups.

### Mutual support and comfort zones

Facilitators were reassured that despite a varied group, people felt able to share things, to discuss differences and use their different strengths for mutual support. Clients were less inhibited than expected when sharing personal information, telling stories and asking questions. Topics that clients found difficult to initiate in one-to-one therapy seemed to be discussed more naturally within the flow of conversation (e.g. sexual relationships, continence), and often introduced humour. The ability to discuss sensitive issues was not an initial aim but was found to be a recurring theme within groups. This identified to the facilitators that the group offered a valuable opportunity to introduce such issues. Once introduced, the more outgoing clients found it easier to expand on the topic, desensitising it for the more reticent clients. The difficulty in bringing these issues to light was how to assist clients in addressing them with relevant family/carers. This highlighted areas for further training and development within the team.

A similar problem arose when discussing feelings and emotions, in that some clients displayed emotionalism and expressed feelings of distress. Fortunately we were able to seek advice from the clinical psychologist attached to the unit, and were given strategies to respond appropriately in future groups. For example, we were advised to allow clients to cry openly, rather than our natural response, which was to stem the upset. The psychologist advised that by inhibiting crying, using methods such as offering tissues or comforting people, we were not allowing clients to release their emotions. The sharing of otherwise distressing issues may have been easier in the group as clients felt less isolated. By realising that other clients were dealing with similar issues it allowed them to 'normalise' the emotions that otherwise they may have considered to be abnormal.

## Equality and participation

The diversity of the group created some practical difficulties in producing supporting material that allowed each member equal access to group discussion. Initially, facilitators found the time required to generate such individualised material and then support the clients in using this within the groups to be taxing. This time constraint reduced over the subsequent groups as facilitators became more familiar with clients' requirements and as a stock of resources was generated. Facilitators felt that it had been unrealistic in aiming to achieve complete equality of participation. A combination of cognitive and communication impairments, emotional responses and premorbid personality created too diverse a range of components to allow true equality. Reflection on this resulted in a more realistic aim for future groups of 'equality of participation by most of the group some of the time'.

## Facilitator management issues

In preparing for the group we had anticipated the support required for clients with cognitive and linguistic impairments but had failed to appreciate the difficulties in managing clients with more pragmatic impairments.

Such clients often dominated groups and did not respond to subtle prompts from facilitators, for example turn taking and inappropriate topics. Initially we tried to deal with this within the group; however, this proved more disruptive and a better solution proved to be addressing it outside the group. In a separate one-to-one session clear boundaries were set and acceptable prompts for use within the group were discussed and agreed upon. While encouraging mutual support among clients, occasions arose where clients offered each other inappropriate advice. In situations where the advice was thought to be detrimental to a client it was necessary to redirect the client to a more suitable solution whilst acknowledging other offers of support.

Although having key themes gave some structure to the group, a level of flexibility was maintained in order for client-led issues to become of equal value to the agenda. The supportive nature of the group and the confidence gained from the collective environment led to an unanticipated management issue. Group members occasionally used this forum to vent their individual frustrations and grievances about daily ward routines, specific incidents or differences of opinions. Although acknowledging the benefit in offloading their negative feelings and thoughts, it posed difficulties for the facilitators in how best to manage this: should it be seen as an opportunity to offload or should a solution be sought? Because, often, the client did not want the issue to be taken further outside the group, a decision was made to continue to allow clients to express themselves this way but to encourage them to think of their own ways of handling these situations in future.

### Practical issues

Problematic practical issues were greater within the first few roll-outs of the group and on initial handover to new facilitators; however, these did reduce over time and as facilitators became familiar with the group and their confidence grew. Preparation and evaluation time was significant initially, especially allocating sufficient time for discussion when completing the VASES and post-group evaluation questionnaire. Although the group itself ran for 90 minutes each week, the amount of time spent doing paperwork, reflections, environment preparation, and handover to team added an extra two hours per week on average dedicated to the group (per facilitator).

The fact that the group was not 'closed' gave more people access to it; however, the practicalities of this meant that the group occasionally felt disjointed and this distracted from complete group cohesion. This placed more demands on the group facilitators to ensure group members were at ease and supported in their participation. In addition, some clients may only have attended two groups prior to discharge from the unit; this required a deal of flexibility from facilitators in allocating time to fit in evaluation sessions prior to their discharge.

The change in facilitators running the group did not result in a greater variance in the measurements obtained from VASES, Non-Sexist Blob Men (Wilson, 1988) and 'Living with Stroke group questionnaire': i.e. similar changes in the range of scores and similar comments in questionnaires were made despite changes in facilitators. Different facilitators experienced and reported similar concerns whilst running the group, which were discussed and resolved outside of the group by the whole team.

## The wider benefits of the group

### For the client

The group provided an opportunity for signposting clients to alternative services (e.g. welfare advice), support groups (e.g. stroke club) and leisure facilities (e.g. accessible holidays). Literature related to topics raised within the groups was provided so clients and careers were able to re-access this when appropriate for them (e.g. lifestyle changes to prevent recurrence of stroke).

Further evidence for clients' benefits was gained through feedback from staff in contact with the clients via the community service following discharge from the unit. After discharge from the unit, many clients who attended the groups maintained friendships made during their stay, and accredited their relationship to attending the group together. Similar results regarding the maintenance of friendships following discharge have been found in studies such as that reported by Elman and Bernstein-Ellis (1999). Community staff reported that clients were less resistant to attending groups held in the community following the running of the 'Living with stroke Group'

### For the team

Staff involved in running the group reported a greater understanding of each other's roles and expertise, in particular cognition and language. This had the greatest impact on the more junior members of the team. The team as a whole developed broader skills in communicating with and supporting all clients with behavioural and emotional issues. Through participating in the group together, staff felt that the relationship they developed with clients was less dependent, and they demonstrated a more active role in their rehabilitation. Staff learned important skills in developing and running a group, particularly flexibility, which allowed the group to be adapted to the needs of the individuals. For example:

- when to prompt
- reassure when necessary
- provide equal opportunity
- acknowledgement that not all clients could have their issues dealt with
- not lecturing
- provide more or less information as required.

**Implications for future groups**

During the running of the group ideas for potential improvements became apparent. Some of these could be incorporated immediately, such as:

- providing 10 minutes for general 'chit chat' to ease into the group;
- to use Likert scales during discussion of topics to assist in measuring the impact on each individual (e.g. pain or sleep);
- a more informal atmosphere could be created by not sitting around a large table (as if in a boardroom meeting);

Other ideas would need to be developed over time, for example:

- The venue used was open to some distraction and interruption; optimally, a room would be required within easy reach of the unit affording greater levels of privacy.
- It was generally acknowledged that the evaluation of the group was not as extensive as it could have been. Various factors influenced the team's capacity to evaluate the group fully, mainly time and an inability to predict all the factors that would require evaluating. For example, the time spent by professionals dealing with clients' emotional issues on a one-to-one basis prior to the group was never measured. That this time was reduced following attendance of the group therefore relied on subjective observations. Although aims for the group were set, it proved difficult to devise a tool to measure whether these had been achieved, in a way in which all clients could participate equally.
- A number of staff felt that benefits would have been gained if a group session could incorporate a visit from past clients. This would give current clients a chance to ask questions about what the future may hold.

## Conclusions

The experiences of those running the group and those participating in it have generally been positive. The aims of the group were realistic and appropriate to the needs of the clients, and the flexibility allowed for individual client-led topics also to be incorporated. The time spent running and evaluating the group was more extensive than anticipated; however, the benefits suggest that it was worthwhile. The Stroke Journey and other visual aids proved to be useful tools and necessary to allow all clients to access the group. All team members had some involvement in the development and running of the group, or at least in discussing its merits/impairments. All staff expressed an interest in making a contribution to the group and gaining a broader understanding of clients' needs and how to address them through their involvement. Subjectively there were great gains to be made from the group; however, in hindsight greater preparation would have allowed for more thorough evaluation to support its benefits. We acknowledge that the diversity and complexity of clients' symptoms made any form of measurement extremely challenging, and feel that the choices made (VASES, Non-Sexist Blob Tree, Living with Stroke group questionnaire) were all useful in measuring change within this client group.

## References

Barton J, Miller A, Chanter J. Emotional adjustment to stroke: a group therapeutic approach. Nursing Times 2002;98:33–35.

Bray M, Todd C. Speech and Language: Clinical Process and Practice. London: Whurr, 2006.

Brumfitt S, Sheeran P. Visual Analogue Self Esteem Scale. Winslow Press, 1999.

Elman RJ, Bernstein-Ellis. Psychosocial aspects of group communication. Treatment Semin Speech Lang 1999;20:65–71.

Kurtz L. Self Help and Support Groups. Thousand Oaks, CA: Sage, 1997.

Luterman, D. Counselling Persons with Communication Disorders and their Families, 3rd edn. Austin, TX: Pro-Ed, 1996.

Markus H, Nurius P. Possible selves. Am Psychol 1986;41:954–969.

Marshall R. Problem focused group therapy for mildly aphasic clients. Am J Speech Lang Pathol 2004;2:31–37.

Royal College of Physicians. National Clinical Guidelines for Stroke, 2nd edn. London: RCP, 2004.

Stroke Association, 2007 (http//:www.stroke.org.uk).

Van Der Gaag A, Smith L, Davis S, Moss B, Cornelius V, Laing S, Mowles C. Therapy and support services for people with long-term stroke and aphasia and their relatives: a six month follow up study. Clin Rehabil 2005;19:372–380.

Wilson P. Games without Frontiers. London: Marshall Pickering, 1988.

Wilson P, Long I. Blob Tree posters. Available from Incentive Plus (www.incentiveplus.co.uk), 2008.

Zigmond AF, Snaith RP. Hospital Anxiety and Depression Scale. Acta Psychiatr Scand 1983; 67:361–370.

## 10 Solution Focused Brief Therapy for People with Acquired Communication Impairments

**Kidge Burns**

## Introduction

Solution Focused Brief Therapy (SFBT) helps clients to see life beyond the problem. Rather than improvement being defined as a reduction in impairment or the promotion of independence, clients have conversations where they are facilitated to find solutions in their immediate situation and environment. As a result clients with mental or physical impairments can see well-being as a balance between themselves as people (the skills and resources that they bring), what they are doing and the environment.

At the Speech and Language Therapy Department in a large acute hospital the solution focused approach has been used over a number of years with many people with acquired communication impairments. It has been demonstrated that many clients are able to determine the timing and number of therapy sessions they attend; numbers of sessions attended now range from one to five, with a few exceptions, and feedback has been positive (Burns, 2005).

This chapter gives a brief outline of SFBT and uses transcripts as part of three case studies to illustrate how clients can think differently and begin to notice what they might be doing to achieve what they want. You will notice a shift in language away from a description of how clients do not want to feel ('depressed' or 'anxious'), to what they are doing when they are 'happy', 'calm' or 'confident'. Their definition of well-being will be unique to themselves, and it is the practitioners' job to facilitate a detailed description of what this looks like in their everyday lives. There is the assumption that knowing the root conditions of clients' impairments is not necessary when building solutions and that 'building solutions is an easier, faster and simpler approach to change in therapy than is problem-solving' (Miller, 2000, p. 28).

## Solution focused brief therapy

Steve de Shazer, born in 1940, was a pioneer in the field of family therapy in Milwaukee and, until his death in 2005, a primary developer in what is now recognised as the SFBT approach. From the mid-1980s he and his wife, Insoo Kim Berg, who died in 2007 aged 72, drew on sources such as Milton Erickson, Buddhism and Ludwig Wittgenstein to develop a minimalist philosophy that has reversed the traditional psychotherapy process of interviewing. Instead of focusing on 'depression', for example, de Shazer is interested in 'non-depression'; those times or exceptions when the problem is absent or less acute, which allow for the practitioner and client to construct a solution (de Shazer, 1994). 'New ideas peculiar to solution focused brief therapy itself include the disconnection between problem and solution, faith in the competence of the client and the lack of a formal theory of change' (Macdonald, 2004).

At BRIEF in London (www.brieftherapy.org.uk) much thought has been given to the 'preferred future' (George, Iveson and Ratner, 1999). In order for therapy to be brief it is important to establish what a preferred future might be and what it might look like; clients are helped to identify ways in which this is already happening and encouraged to look for signs that further change might occur. Getting a description of the preferred future rather than starting with exceptions means that the conversation 'will relate specifically to what the clients want to happen in the future' (George, Iveson and Ratner, 2006, p. 14). Solution focused practitioners do this by inviting clients to view their lives 'through a number of theoretical lenses: cognitive, linguistic, behavioural, narrative, experiential and systemic' (George, Iveson and Ratner, 2006, p. 24). The idea that a therapist should aim to 'intervene' as little as possible in clients' lives, so as to give more room to the client's voice, is central to the solution focused practice.

## Preferred futures

A medical classification of diagnoses alone tends to focus us on the physical rather than the functional or psychological impact of a disease. Rather than spend time linking a specific type of intervention to a specific problem and describing what they are doing, therapists need to focus on how they are facilitators in reducing the impact of a condition on a client's life and how this can be measured in some way. It is particularly important to establish clients' 'best hopes' in the first session as 'it seems commonsense that if you know where you want to go, then getting there is easier' (de Shazer et al., 1986, p. 213). Clients will talk about outcomes if we ask them 'What are your best hopes from this session/conversation?'

Peter is 64 and has had Parkinson's disease (PD) for over 15 years. He comes to the hospital in a wheelchair with his wife Silvia (not their real names) to see if he can 'speak more clearly'. The speech and language therapist (SLT) could focus on times when speech is more intelligible, but this is the first session and she is interested in a description of the preferred future. She asks the Miracle Question (MQ), perceived by many to be 'a central intervention in the solution focused repertoire' (O'Connell and Palmer, 2003):

'Now, I want to ask you a strange question. Suppose that while you are sleeping tonight and the entire house is quiet, a miracle happens. The miracle is that the problem which brought you here is solved. However, because you are sleeping, you don't know that the miracle has happened. So, when you wake up tomorrow morning, what will be different that will tell you that a miracle has happened and the problem which brought you here is solved?' (de Shazer, 1988, p. 5).

The 'miracle' is not that the Parkinson's disease has gone but that communication may have improved (Peter's best hopes) and he is able to identify some changes directly related to this; the picture expands to include more than the stated goal. The MQ helps him identify 'little things [that] make life easier', such as his DIY, and he acknowledges that sometimes he knows better than others what to do, enabling him to see times when he has more control over his life.

The next part of the session involves Silvia in the experience of imagining a time when change is happening and what difference that might make in her interaction with Peter. The value of seeing people together is that people who are part of a system can influence each other; systemic or 'other person perspective' questions invite Silvia to use language that suggests alternative possibilities to the situation at home.

English is not her first language and the therapist finds that frequent repetition and rephrasing appears to aid understanding.

| | |
|---|---|
| **Therapist** | What would tell you that things had moved on a little bit in terms of communication generally? What would be one thing you would notice that would make a difference? Little thing ... it doesn't have to be that big picture tomorrow. What one little thing would have to happen? |
| **Silvia** | Um ... (*pause*) What shall I say now? (*turning to Peter*) Sometimes he gets so frustrate, frustrate, cause I didn't understand him, you know. And I want his improvement on that. |
| **T** | Okay, that sounds ... you know ... So instead of being frustrated Peter will be ... what? What would you notice, instead of being frustrated? He would be ...? |
| **S** | Well ... more calmed down, you know. |
| **T** | Okay, so suppose he was a little more calmed down. What would you notice him doing differently? |
| **S** | (*pause*) I'm not intelligent person. I don't know. |

| T | I think that's a lovely example. It's exactly the example that I think is useful because you're saying . . . you're quite right, it's not just the speaking . . . it's the whole, when we communicate, the whole thing. And you're saying he would be calmer. So how would you know? What would you notice that would tell you that Peter is calm, not getting frustrated? |
| S | I'd see . . . on him. You know, the way he's talking or the way, you know, the way he calls me or whatever. |
| T | So how would he be calling you? |
| S | Not always, but you know sometimes . . . er . . . we get fed up. |
| T | Of course. So he'd be . . . |
| S | I shouting and . . . he's shouting and when he's shouting it's . . . well, I cannot understand nothing at all. |

Using the phrase and complimenting Silvia on the 'calmed down' idea, the therapist believes Silvia will find her way through the 'noticing' question, with a little encouragement! This is done in the belief that it will highlight and make explicit Silvia's resources. Difficulties will be acknowledged and normalised, but the therapist will keep going with the future focus in order to help the conversation shift from a problem-focused description to a more solution focused one. However, as solution focused practitioners such as Guy Shennan point out, while retaining a focus in our work we also need to allow for our future focus to be more than a set of rigid goals and that equally important is a sense of 'developing a generally forward momentum towards various, more desired ways of living' (O'Connell and Palmer, 2003, p. 43).

| T | Okay, so suppose that . . . you noticed Peter was a bit calmer, what would you notice that . . . how that was happening? What would he be doing that would tell you? You're saying that he would call you differently? |
| S | I think so. Maybe. I don't know. |
| T | In what way? |
| S | I'll going to understand better. I dunno. Or hear better. |
| T | And what else? How else would you know that he was calmer? It might be nothing to do with speaking. |
| S | Oh, I can see on his face. |
| T | Aha. What do you see? |
| S | You know . . . when he, um . . . and when he's calm his face is relax . . . yeah. |

| | |
|---|---|
| T | Aha. Like now? |
| S | Yeah. But he's get a little bit tired. I can see, when he try to speak. |
| T | Okay. Well I've been asking lots of funny questions so . . . its very tiring! *(laughing)* You've been very patient. So . . . it's . . . you're right. It's about, erm, seeing in somebody's face, which if you know each other very well you see instantly that somebody is calmer. And what difference . . . if you saw that more, what difference would that make to you? What would you be doing differently if you saw that calm face? |
| S | Maybe I'll come calmer too, you know. |
| T | Ahhh. |
| S | *(laugh)* |
| T | So . . . what would you be doing if that happened, if you were a bit calmer? |
| S | Erm, well maybe we understand much better. |
| T | Aha. |
| S | I don't know. |
| T | Yeah. I think it's possible, isn't it. When we're calmer . . . I mean it makes a difference, doesn't it. |
| S | Umm. |
| T | So . . . *(turning to Peter)* suppose she was being calmer. What would you notice her doing differently? |

The conversation has reinforced Silvia's 'expert' knowledge of her husband and created a visual picture, translating a feeling into something observable. Exploring the scenario further from Peter's perspective the therapist stays with the visual image of them behaving in a different way with each other. 'These different responses can come to serve as reinforcements for the client's different behaviours, thus also reinforcing the inner changes' (Miller and de Shazer, 1998, p. 366). The focus moves from just looking at the communication to how the future might look generally if things were different.

A solution focused approach reminds the therapist to keep looking for the couple's skills, resources and common goals. It is questionable whether any SLT exercises can help Peter, although he is given various handouts at the end of the session regarding communication. Before using SFBT the therapist would have spent therapy time going through these handouts, although they are largely self-explanatory. Now, however, they are able to have a conversation that looks at Peter's life through a wider description of events than just the immediate impact of PD.

Silvia is also invited to think of future change and her coping skills are acknowledged. It is noticeable in the video recording of this session that the atmosphere between them changes, and Silvia admits that she has never spoken about the situation in such a way before: 'The way I talk to you I never told him'.

Talking about an 'easier', 'calmer' life, Peter's speech has become more intelligible. Most SLTs will know that if people are relaxed and feeling 'well' in themselves there is a chance they might be speaking more slowly and that this in turn can facilitate communication. If clients can demonstrate this for themselves then information has been gathered in a collaborative way and the handouts, rather than 'teach' relaxation or improved breath support, merely reinforce client expertise and understanding of what they are already doing.

Peter asks for an appointment in 2 months time but he is unable to make this appointment and to date he has been seen for only one session.

In the first session considerable time can be spent on exploring the picture of the preferred future, but describing the future does not mean that clients have to be tied to specific goals. Clients may become more aware of signs of how they want their lives to be in the time between sessions, when they are living their everyday lives, rather than in the session itself. With Peter and Silvia the therapist keeps the conversation in the future so as to elicit multiple possible signs of the preferred future. At BRIEF, the idea of 'Gallery One & Two' (Iveson, personal communication, 2006) sees this process as looking at a picture in detail and then going to the next room, rather than constantly changing from one room to the next, which risks losing the 'flow' and 'theme' of what is on show. Gallery One has pictures of the preferred future whereas Gallery Two has pictures of the past and present, where some of this preferred future may already be happening. In the latter, the solution focused practitioner moves on to questions such as 'What parts of this "miracle" are already happening in your life?'

### Preferred future questions

- Suppose this miracle happened, what would you be doing differently?
- What one thing would you notice that would make a difference?
- Instead of being frustrated you/X would be . . . what?
- How would you know?
- What would you notice X doing?
- What else?
- What difference would that make?

## Signs of the preferred future already happening

Kristy is 40 and is admitted to hospital with multiple sclerosis (MS) and expressive dysphasia. After discharge she returns to the hospital as an outpatient and is seen by a SLT and her student. Part of the first session is undertaken by the student, who conducts a formal assessment to look at word-finding difficulties.

Critics of the solution focused approach comment on the 'neglect of client history and broader assessment' (Stalker, Levene and Coady, 1999, p. 473) and that the giving of information is avoided, as this would cast the therapist in the role of the expert (Kerr, 2001). With regard to the latter, this can be addressed by the way in which the information is given (if it is specifically requested) and that handouts can be taken home if necessary, so that clients can decide how useful they might be in their own time.

With Kristy there is much talk about 'loss of confidence', 'loss of control' and 'embarrassment'. The SLT asks her client about her best hopes and by the end of the first session there is a list of Kristy's strengths and resources that she has been using to manage her life since leaving hospital. A solution focused practitioner can know more about a client's life than the referrer within a brief period of time, without the need for a lengthy case history or 'broader assessment'. Scales are one of the questioning frameworks that facilitate this.

In SFBT the scale framework, generally used on a 0 to 10 basis, enables clients to rate themselves in terms of where they are in relation to their preferred future at 10 and how they have managed to keep from 0. The scale can be a visual record where clients mark themselves on a line between 0 and 10 with added pictures of faces or diagrams if there is a difficulty with understanding.

Rather than rate the problem (which, if it is only related to speech, for example, may or may not improve), the SLT will introduce scales after clients have described their preferred future; 10 can then represent a number of different possibilities, which frequently include descriptions of a sense of well-being. Scales also facilitate people to settle for a number, which is lower than 10, as 'good enough'.

Kristy is asked: 'Imagine a scale from 0 to 10 with 10 representing your best hopes are achieved and 0 being the opposite of this. Where would you say you are now?'

Initially Kristy gives herself 3–4 (where 10 = control and energy in her life), and the following week she feels things have improved, so that she is able to rate herself as 5.5. The reasons she gives for this are:

1. she feels supported by the SLT and more confident in her knowledge of MS;
2. she is more aware of her limitations regarding her 2-hour limit on activity before she fatigues and she is able to pace herself better than when they first met
3. she is taking ginkgo biloba.

She is given another scale where 10 = she is very confident she can improve on this first scale, and 0 = the opposite; she feels she is currently at 5–6.

Working with these two scales a solution focused practitioner can help clients to describe things that they have already done, as well as what they might do to move further up the scale. If the numbers are low on the scales it can be useful to look at how clients have managed to be above 0 or to explore other areas of their lives that have not suffered. Alternatively, it may be useful to stay with examining how clients have managed to cope in such a difficult situation.

Even if 10 is perceived to be unachievable by various professionals, there seems to be something about the process of working with scales that helps clients become more confident about what they have already achieved and to look for small signs that will tell them further progress has occurred. Fortunately there is growing awareness in the field of speech and language therapy that 'self-report measures are able to encompass a holistic view of the disorder and test therapy's mettle outside the confines of the clinic [and] the clinician' expectations' (Guntupalli, Kalinowski and Saltuklaroglu, 2006, p. 4).

The first session initiates a search for the client's preferred future: whether the search has been successful or not it 'would lead predictably to the next step' (de Shazer, 1988, p. 63). The follow-up sessions will begin with 'What's better?' or 'What have you been pleased to notice since we last met?' as the assumption in SFBT is that clients may have noticed improvements since the first meeting. In the third session Kristy continues to notice positive changes in her life and that she has, on occasions, been at a 7 on her first scale.

The following transcript comes from the fourth session when, in response to 'What's better?' Kristy tells the therapist about how she has managed to buy and install a new computer.

| | |
|---|---|
| **Therapist** | So you got the Mac and you've done it in a couple of days. |
| **Kristy** | Yeah, actually I'm up and running. |
| T | So how does that feel? |
| K | A huge relief. Enormous relief. Actually that . . . that might have been a moment of epiphany. That might have been an 8. |
| T | Hey! |
| K | Just because I couldn't send anything to anyone last week until it started running. Then it started running. And I could send the e-mails out and get it going. |
| T | Gosh. |
| K | It's nice to be creative. It's a different part of my brain as well. I feel it and that helps. I think it's what I'm supposed to be doing, kind of thing. I need to work. |
| T | So that moment of 8 . . . that epiphany. What . . . what did you do differently? |

K    I think I allowed myself to...to momentarily revel in the moment of...of...it was a very relaxing and relief-making feeling that something was working for a change.

T    So what were you doing that told you...you were feeling...

K    *(interrupts)* It was that moment when I finally, finally received...it sounds very small, but when I received an e-mail, because X had received her e-mail. Because for days it wasn't working. And suddenly it's like 'THIS IS WORKING'. It was like 'This is good'. Which is good. It was nice. Silly...

T    And who else saw that? I mean, your husband?

K    Nobody. I told him later. But he's a computer buff, he knows all this stuff, so to him it's like using a fork; 'What's the big deal?' But this is not easy for him because he feels—I can only imagine—pressured by the whole thing, having to carry the weight of the world on his shoulders and he's not at that point in his life where he feels like he wants to work through these things and find ways of expressing. It just 'is' and 'I'm getting on with it' kind of thing. That's what he's doing.

T    So...I mean, over the past week. What tells you that...you know, I see what you're saying about you're the one who's having to live with this right now...what erm...signs are there that he might be dealing with it just a tiny bit better than he was before? I mean one thing that tells you that?

K    Oh...erm...

T    ...that he sees you getting on with things, that maybe he's...

K    Yeah, he...he...when he married me I was in the middle of a million jobs and a million different things. Maybe on Sunday night...um...I'd worked all day Saturday and then X really needed to see some of the work before she went away. And he was very cool about that. And he just said 'Yeah, go! I know. I know you have to go'. We were supposed to have roast dinner and he said 'Don't worry, I'll slam the duck in'. He saved me some. So that was a nice moment. He's very, he's very cool about me going and doing my work because that's how he likes me because it takes the pressure off him to feel he's the only one who's breadwinning. Yeah.

T    So that sounds good.

K    Yeah. Yeah. Actually not bad. It's certainly getting there. Slowly. Bit by bit.

You will notice that the therapist stays with the moment of Kristy achieving her 'epiphany'. Kristy is able to compliment herself on being creative, which is probably more meaningful than if the therapist had paid her the compliment. Kristy has previously described the strained relationship she has been having with her husband since the diagnosis of MS, and the therapist is curious about change since the last session. The cooked duck seems to be an event that is significant to Kristy; through answering the therapist's questions she is beginning to put into words a clearer description of a positive past and present and displaying her ability to interpret aspects of her social system that are working effectively. As with so many clients 'things become clearer as they try to articulate something they have been only vaguely aware of' (Berg and Dolan, 2001, p. 80).

There is a gap of nearly 4 months between the fourth and fifth sessions. Kristy says that she has memory lapses and ongoing difficulties with her language but that she has been able to talk about her condition in her workplace. She is determined 'not to feel afflicted, the victim...' and when asked what she would like to feel instead she identifies this as being 'more in control'. Interestingly, although she feels she is less 'in control' with her husband she has noticed 'he seems more fond of me'. What tells her that? 'There are more cuddles'.

### Follow-up questions

- What's been better? What have you been pleased to notice?
- What did you do differently?
- Who else saw that?
- Over the past week/month what signs are there that X might be dealing with things differently?
- What tells you that?

Kristy tells the therapist that she feels she's 'doing alright' and would like to leave the door open regarding another session. If she has not contacted the department after 3 months she will be discharged, based on the assumption that her needs have been met in some way and that she will contact the department again if she wants to.

A report will be sent to her doctor, formulated in a solution focused way, in the knowledge that although many SLTs work within a problem-focused community it is possible to hear the opinions of everyone involved in a case and then 'respectfully combine (and sometimes reword) these into a useful professional recommendation' (Pichot and Dolan, 2003, p. 135).

## Closing sessions

Following on from a presentation on SFBT to some consultants and their medical teams, two referrals are sent to the SLT department for further input. Both have had previous help for their speech and language as well as help from various other therapists/counsellors in an attempt to alleviate some of the distress that these individuals are experiencing as a result of a stroke. Both talk of wanting 'to end it all'.

One of these individuals is Jane, a woman of 45 who is referred with 'mild receptive and expressive dysphasia affecting spoken and written words as a result of a right temporo-parietal infarct in June 2005'.

SFBT can be helpful to clients even if they have difficulties with abstract reasoning, memory, language processing or reduced attention span. Respectful of clients' views of their own lives, the practitioner can work with anyone who can have a conversation, however brief. Naturally, this may involve repetition, concrete examples and language that reflects the clients' frame of reference—something the solution focused practitioner is already good at!

Another established part of SFBT is to end the session with a brief summary of what has appeared significant to the client; this may be something useful that clients are already doing towards achieving their preferred future or coping skills that they show in dealing with their situation. Practitioners usually take a break and leave the room so as to construct a message that best reflects what has been discussed in the session. Even if there has been a lot of 'problem talk' it is always possible to give an affirmation of what clients are hoping to see as different in the future and a reminder as to how this has been discussed in the session. This is particularly useful for clients who may have difficulty with cognitive processing and recall. There is evidence that unsuccessful therapists tend to focus on their clients' impairments rather than their strengths, and that when they do focus on their clients' strengths at the end of a session it is too late to have a positive effect. Successful therapists, on the other hand, focus on their clients' strengths from the very start of a therapy session and make sure they end sessions by returning to their clients' strengths (Gassman and Grawe, 2006).

When talking about the preferred future Jane was initially focused on a return to her previous life, but 2 years after her stroke it is unlikely, for example, that she will be able to return to the job she had before. She needs to set herself new goals for the future, but in the past others have given her ideas and suggestions that she has been unable or unwilling to carry through. Identifying that her confidence is low, Jane now spends time in the sessions (and more importantly, between the sessions) noticing what she is already doing that gives her ' . . . a reason for living. I was a very positive person. I can't go on being so negative'.

Jane may have had a stroke but she still has strengths and resources that she brings from the past. The practitioner's job is to help her focus more on this area of her life as well as being sensitive to the difficulties she encounters. Comments such as 'I was a very positive person' invite the question 'So what do you notice yourself doing now that tells you that you can still be positive?' 'What does your husband notice you doing that tells him this? 'If you were to rate yourself as 10 = as positive as you could possibly be and 0 = the opposite, where would you mark yourself on this line (*marked out on paper*)?'

The last question, asked in session three, was answered with 'I'm three-quarters [up the scale]. I can see that I can remember names now which is good'. Jane's husband was sitting next to her and appeared surprised by this response—answers can sometimes be unexpected to the therapist, clients and their partners. Jane may still talk about 'today is a dying day' but these comments are less frequent and she is noticing signs of change: 'There hasn't been a dramatic change but a little bit—that's enough for now. I see things differently. I am special.'

Jane's husband feels she needs 'more confidence'. Here again the solution focused approach helps to translate inner states into outward criteria; in response to 'What difference will that make to you if she is a bit more confident?' he answers 'She needs to talk to me more', and Jane says 'I know I can do that'.

Clearly it is 'not easy to put aside our highly valued urge to look behind and beneath, to understand and to explain things, and thus to just describe what happens' (Berg and de Shazer, 1993, p. 22). SFBT encourages the practitioner to be 'minimal'—to keep out of our clients' lives and give them and their ideas as much space as possible, as opposed to formulating our own ideas as to how change occurs (George, Iveson and Ratner, 2001).

At the end of every session the therapist asks Jane 'What have you found useful about the session?' (as opposed to 'Have you found the session useful?'). This question is based on the assumption that clients can highlight material for themselves before they leave and that it is useful to both client and therapist to know that they are moving together in the right direction:

**Therapist**   Maybe you'd like to tell me how you've found it useful coming.

**Jane**   Um. I think it's just . . . um . . . having somebody outside the situation who hasn't got, who hasn't got anything too absorbing about . . . about this to know what, what . . . erm . . . they think about what I'm gaining and what I'm achieving. And so that, that's the difference. Because I don't, I don't feel that I'm achieving anything. But I have to . . . I do listen to what you say . . . err . . . if you said something then I would . . . erm . . . I would try and do it, even if I couldn't. You don't, you don't . . . erm . . . you don't push me on anything but you do . . . do say that I should, I should do something. You feel that I should do something. And I would do it. And . . . um . . . that would be err . . . more meaningful to me.

T        Aha. I mean I suppose the thing is that I don't know what's
         going to be meaningful to you or give you that sense of
         achievement. The only person—as even maybe your hus-
         band doesn't know, I don't know—but probably the person
         who *is* going to notice it, even if it's the smallest thing is
         going to be you and I think that thing of noticing ... that
         you're obviously thinking about it and noticing.

J        Yeah. I suppose I could try a little bit more. I could think
         about things a little bit more, but I don't, I don't know
         whether it'll be worth it. I'll try it though.

T        Yeah? Okay. Good. That sounds good to me.

Notice how the therapist's language reflects that of the client. The
therapist is not always 100% sure what Jane is trying to say but she has
a sense that Jane is giving these conversations a lot of thought and that
this appears to be meaningful. The therapist accepts Wittgenstein's idea
that the different uses of language are like paths that take us in different
directions and that if everything is there on the surface of things then
(regardless of Jane's current behaviour or level of fluency), her language
suggests that there are signs of change. Jane may not be able to speak or
do things as she did before but she might be seeing a change in how she
is dealing with things and this change could be the difference that makes
a difference. 'A solution focused approach to health adopts a "holistic"
stance that links body, mind and spirit with the social environment'
(O'Connell, 2005, p. 137).

The solution focused practitioner assumes that clients are experts in
knowing what is or is not useful to them. It is logical, therefore, to ask
clients if they want to come back.

T        So would it be useful for you to come again? What do you think?

J        It would be useful for me to come again but if it's alright with
         you. Because um ... I have to think about it for a long time and to
         do ... do something to make it more practical.

T        Okay. I like the sound of that.

J        Um ... I have to do it but I can't. But I have to try very very hard.

T        I think it's going to be hard work. I think you're right. I think
         you're absolutely right.

J        Do you think I've improved my ... erm ... my speech since I've
         been coming to see you?

T        I think your speaking when you first came was pretty good.
         You've got a fantastic use of vocabulary which I'm constantly
         thinking 'Ooooh, that's a nice way of putting things'. I suspect
         you've always had that probably?

| J | Yeah, she mentioned it in . . . in Italy . . . my friend. Yeah. |
|---|---|
| T | Really? So other people are noticing that! |
| J | Yeah. Um . . . she said it was . . . um . . . it was very specific and very dogmatic . . . the way I . . . I said things that were very um . . . clear for her. Yeah. |
| T | Yeah. Right, well it's great other people are noticing that, isn't it? |

Jane values the opinion of the SLT regarding her speech and it would be churlish to refuse to give feedback on the grounds that the therapist should avoid giving any 'expert' opinion. However, she uses it as an opportunity to link in to Jane's past communication skills; as a result the conversation moves out again to a wider context and a comment from a friend, given when Jane and her husband were visiting Italy the previous week.

Jane decides on another appointment and leaves with the task of continuing to notice what might be 'meaningful' to her. This 'noticing' type suggestion is an attempt to keep therapeutic suggestions to a minimum (George, Iveson and Ratner, 2003). There is no specific goal given to Jane that she *has* to do. As it happens the next session reveals that she has indeed thought about 'talking more' to her husband and he is delighted that on one particular evening she chats to him on the sofa for a while (when on other occasions he says this would not have happened). Jane says 'I had to make a decision'.

Is this a change in 'well-being'? Jane's husband reports that she seems happier in herself since the first appointment and the therapist is confident that there will be further signs of progress when they next meet.


## Outcome

> Contrary to the commonsense view, change is seen to happen *within* language: What we talk about and how we talk about it makes a difference, and it is such differences that can be used to make a difference (to the client). Thus reframing a 'marital problem' into an 'individual problem' or an 'individual problem' into a 'marital problem' makes a difference both in how we talk about things and in where we look for solutions
>
> *de Shazer (1994, p. 10)*

In all three case examples given in this chapter, the effects of acquired communication impairments are noticed within the individuals' relationship with their spouse. We could see the impairments as 'marital' impairments requiring specialist help from therapists trained to deal with couples. Similarly we could see specific impairments related to specific communication difficulties or look at the 'severity' of the impairment and whether it has occurred as a single event or as a result of chronic disease. Trying to link specific techniques to a specific diagnosis can be unhelpful; SFBT is an approach that encourages change and one that assumes that there are more similarities than differences between these individuals.

Some therapists can stay with one model rather than integrate others because a meta-theory requires us in some way to assess our client; 'we will have to move outside the solution focused frame to do so and at that point a solution focused approach is likely to falter' (Iveson, personal communication, 2005). Others may work in agency settings that require them to work with bereavement or trauma, for example, in a particular way. In an environment that is not based on SFBT, solution focused practitioners need to look for the common ground with colleagues, rather than the differences.

It is helpful to apply the same questions to ourselves as to the clients when approaching any potential areas of conflict: 'How are you already bringing solution focused thinking into your agency role and tasks?' 'Suppose your work with other professionals and agencies was as cooperative and effective as it could be—what would it look like?' The point here is that we need to pay attention to our own well-being and have the opportunity to use the solution focused framework to facilitate our own thinking. This allows us to appreciate its effectiveness, which will in turn have a bearing on our own clients.

When a whole department has been trained in SFBT there can be a commitment, for example, to allow the clients to determine when they want to return for the next session or whether they no longer need to be seen (rather than committing clients to a package, say, of six sessions). Even if clients are being seen as inpatients, we can work with them or their carers in a way that is respectful of their wishes allowing, of course, for any professional requirements regarding risk management.

One perceived difficulty in dealing with psychological well-being is that therapy input will be never-ending. Take the example of Jane, who has been seen now for seven sessions over a period of 6 months. She is still noticing progress with her speech and language but the main concerns around her confidence level and coping skills are ongoing. The SLT will extend the gaps between the sessions as much as possible so as to encourage her to notice signs of progress, our primary concern being effectiveness rather than dependence on the therapist. Questions can help with this, and some examples are offered here:

'If 10 = we don't need to meet any more, and 0 = how things were when you made arrangements to come here, where are you now?'
'Suppose it's the time when you'll be discharged, what will you be doing?'
'How will your partner/best friend/dog notice that things have become better?

As mentioned at the beginning of the chapter, findings suggest that we can reduce the length of therapy input with all client groups as a result of working with SFBT. Similar findings were reported in de Shazer's summary of Milwaukee outcome studies in 1991 (Miller, Hubble and Duncan, 1996), which have been reflected in subsequent studies (McDonald, 2007). A number of therapists follow the criterion that regardless of the nature or severity of the problem each case is limited to a maximum of 10 one-hour sessions (Weakland, Fisch, Watzlawick and Boding, 1974). Experience has shown that with a person like Jane it would be appropriate to end therapy after 10 to 12 sessions; scales would be one way of measuring progress and establishing the signs that will tell her we no longer need to meet. Hence the importance of negotiating what the outcome of therapy will look like and being clear about what the client can realistically achieve in therapy.

On discharge, it is required practice to write a letter to the referrer, a copy of which is now sent to the client. Report writing will change as a result of SFBT: a report on the single session with Peter, for example, includes a reminder of how well he is doing on his scales (he scales how well he feels he can improve on communication at home, for example, and marks himself at 6/7), and it also includes compliments to Silvia, with examples she gives that testify to her coping skills.

## Conclusions

The therapist is client-led and the basic assumptions remain the same. The first session will start by focusing on what clients want from therapy followed by what they have done in the past or what they are doing now that links in with the preferred future. It will end with what signs they might notice regarding further progress. Second or subsequent sessions focus on exploring change, highlighting progress and looking for the next small signs of progress. The essence of SFBT is:

- to see a person as being more than their problem;
- to look for resources rather than deficits;
- to explore possible and preferred futures;
- to explore what is already contributing to those futures;
- and to treat clients as the experts in all aspects of their lives (George, Iveson and Ratner, 2006, p. 2).

Clients talk about their belief that having conversations about hope and change (rather than despair and feeling 'stuck'), generate feelings that affect physiology and symptoms. Take the example of Robert McCrum, in his book 'My Year Off: Rediscovering Life After A Stroke'. He comments: 'I have come to believe that by stressing normality and activity the stroke-sufferer has a better chance of recovery. The brain and its workings remain a mystery to doctors, but I am certain that adopting a vigorous and positive attitude to recovery actually assists the process of renewal. I cannot prove this; it's what I believe to have been true in my own case' (McCrum, 1998, p. 217).

We cannot know from the diagnosis how clients view their own recovery or what they wish to accomplish. It is imperative, therefore, that we ask our clients in the first session what their best hopes are from the admission/session/conversation. Fortunately the Department of Health recognises the importance of 'The Expert Patient', and in areas such as chronic disease there is now emphasis on 'research and practical experience in North America and Britain [which] are showing that today's patients with chronic diseases need not be mere recipients of care. They can become key decision-makers in the treatment process' (Department of Health, 2001).

SFBT provides us with questions that enable us to work with clients as briefly as possible; conversations range from 10 minutes on the ward (where attention span is sometimes difficult to maintain) to 1-hour sessions. Other professionals such as doctors, who. need to conduct appointments within a tight time frame, find this aspect of a solution focused approach especially useful (Unwin, 2005).

In the national clinical guidelines for stroke there is talk of 'one of the characteristics of rehabilitation is the setting of goals... [and] the perceptions of service users are an important way of evaluating service delivery' (Royal College of Physicians, 2004). The way scales are used in SFBT facilitates this, particularly as they are drawn up by the clients without rigid adherence to numbers or specified 'steps'. The language of the solution focused practitioner reflects this: 'What would be a *sign* that things are changing/that you're maintaining this situation as you would like?' 'What are the signs of hope that things will get better?' Change may be small and may not reach 10 on a scale but in hospital particularly, or after a period of time when things appear to plateau, another number may be recognised as 'good enough'.

By exploring change and highlighting progress through the perspective of the other person, clients are helped to see change in a wider context. Kristy found this especially useful: 'What has your husband/colleagues/child noticed?' 'Who else has noticed?' Clients move from talking about a sense of what is 'right' for them to thinking about 'doing' it. By answering questions such as these they are likely to notice more when the 'doing' is already happening.

Another outcome of these questions is represented by the concrete examples of clients' activities that can be documented in medical notes, case conferences and reports. Rather than endless documentation of the problem from another professional, evidence suggests that medical teams are often more interested in this focus on solutions. Because the impact of a condition can be measured on a self-rating scale, outcomes and reflective tools, such as Kate Malcomess' Care Aims (Anderson and Van der Gaag, 2005), fit in comfortably with SFBT.

The solution focused practitioner asks questions to facilitate clients to gather more information on how they are managing their situation. With time clients are able to ask the questions themselves, such as 'What difference did that make?' and 'What else did I notice?' and take active steps to notice change within themselves and their environment, thereby becoming less reliant on 'help' from a professional. The opportunities within SFBT to compliment and to generate self compliments enhance the well-being of solution focused practitioners and clients alike.

The questions we ask influence what clients notice. SFBT has been described as simple but not easy; when they meet with professionals, clients can feel they are expected to talk at length about 'the problem', especially if there is the perception that, if they sound too 'well', the support systems will be withdrawn before they feel ready. The solution focused practitioner follows the client lead as to what they want to do in a session and uses solution focused questions to facilitate this. If the situation is perceived as being particularly difficult then an acknowledgement of the effort that is required to keep going may be all that is possible. This is certainly the case when Jane is first seen.

No solution focused practitioner is going to be solution 'forced', and it is always apparent in any video recordings of SFBT that the client feels listened to. Watching SFBT in practice reminds us of how important it is to reflect on our own use of language rather than the mechanics of the questions.

Wittgenstein and Steve de Shazer see language as a game where words are defined by the context in which they are used. It is up to us to invite clients such as Peter, Kristy and Jane to describe a preferred future and explore change in the past or the present so that 'they come to believe in the truth or reality of what they are talking about. This is the way language works, naturally' (Berg and de Shazer, 1993, p. 9).

## References

Anderson C, Van der Gaag A (eds). Speech and Language Therapy: Issues in Professional Practice. London: Whurr Publishers, 2005.

Berg IK, Dolan Y. Tales of Solutions: A Collection of Hope-Inspiring Stories. New York: Norton, 2001

Berg IK, de Shazer S. Making numbers talk: language in therapy. In: Steven F (ed.) The New Language of Change: Constructive Collaboration in Psychotherapy. New York: Guilford Press, 1993.

Burns K. Focus on Solutions: a Health Professional's Guide. London: Whurr Publishers, 2005.

Department of Health. The Expert Patient: a New Approach to Chronic Disease Management for the 21st Century. London: Department of Health, 2001.

de Shazer S. Clues: Investing Solutions in Brief Therapy. New York: Norton, 1988.

de Shazer S. Words were Originally Magic. New York: Norton, 1994.

de Shazer S, Berg IK, Lipchik E, Nunnally E, Molnar A, Gingerich W, Weiner-Davis M. Brief therapy: focused solution development. Family Process 1986;25:207–222.

Gassman D, Grawe K. General change mechanisms: The relation between problem activation and resource activation in successful and unsuccessful therapeutic interactions. Clin Psychol Psychother 2006;13:1–11.

George E, Iveson C, Ratner H. Problem to Solution: Brief Therapy with Individuals and Families. London: Brief Therapy Press, 1999.

George E, Iveson C, Ratner H. Sharpening Ockham's razor. Paper delivered at EBTA conference, Dublin, 2001.

George E, Iveson C, Ratner H. Beyond solutions. Paper delivered at EBTA conference, Berlin, 2003.

George E, Iveson C, Ratner H. BRIEFER: a Solution Focused Manual. London: BRIEF, 2006.

Guntupalli VK, Kalinowski J, Saltuklaroglu T. The need for self-report data in the assessment of stuttering therapy efficacy: repetitions and prolongations of speech. The stuttering syndrome. Int J Lang Comm Dis 2006;41:1–18.

Kerr L. An assessment of adaptability to feminist principles of solution focused brief therapy as practised by Insoo Kim Berg. J Syst Ther 2001;20:77–99.

Macdonald A. Solution focused practice: existing competencies and preferred futures. UKASFP Conference, Preston, 2004.

Macdonald A. Solution focused Therapy: Theory, Research and Practice. London: Sage, 2007.

McCrum R. My Year Off: Rediscovering Life After A Stroke. London: Picador, 1998.

Miller G. From "how" to "what" questions. Ratkes 2/ 2000: 24–29.

Miller G, de Shazer S. Have you heard the latest rumour about . . . ? Solution focused therapy as a rumour. Family Process 1998;37:363–377.

Miller S, Hubble M, Duncan B. Handbook of Solution Focused Brief Therapy. San Francisco: Jossey-Bass, 1996.

O'Connell B. Solution focused Therapy, 2nd edn. London: Sage, 2005.

O'Connell B, Palmer S (eds). Handbook of Solution focused Therapy. London: Sage, 2003.

Pichot T, Dolan Y. Solution focused Brief Therapy: its Effective Use in Agency Settings. New York: Haworth, 2003.

Royal College of Physicians. National Clinical Guidelines for Stroke, 2nd edn. London: Royal College of Physicians, 2004.

Stalker C, Levene J, Coady N. Solution focused brief therapy—one model fits all? Families in Society: the Journal of Contemporary Human Services 1999;80:468–477.

Unwin D. SFGP! Why a solution focused approach is brilliant in primary care. Solution News 2005;1:10–12.

Weakland J, Fisch R, Watzlawick P, Boding A. Brief therapy: focused problem resolution. Family Process 1974;12:141–168.

# Index

Note: page numbers in *italics* refer to figures.